1991

Birth Ethics

Birth Ethics

RELIGIOUS AND CULTURAL VALUES IN THE GENESIS OF LIFE

Kenneth L. Vaux

CROSSROAD · NEW YORK

1989

The Crossroad Publishing Company
370 Lexington Avenue, New York, N.Y. 10017

Printed in the United States of America

Library of Congress Cataloging-in-Publication Data

Vaux, Kenneth L., 1939–
    Birth ethics : religious and cultural values in the genesis of
life / Kenneth L. Vaux.
        p.   cm.
    Bibliography: p.
    Includes index.
    ISBN 0-8245-0955-2
    1. Medical ethics. 2. Medicine—Religious aspects—Christianity.
I. Title.
R725.55.V38   1989   89-7825
176—dc20   CIP

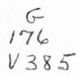

Contents

Preface

PILGRIMAGE

One's art is a resurrection, whether it be musical composition, painting, or manuscript. Something dead or dormant has been brought to life. Unlike the divine creation, this creation may be faltering or uncomely, but it is manifest, it lives. In this sense any creative work is incarnation, resurrection, and life. Like the Lazarus of Eugene O'Neill, it may be hounded into its tomb with raucous laughter; or like Sylvia Plath's *Lady Lazarus*, it may expire in the mouth of the oven, the flaming red hair now lying limp, its only vital reminiscence. Despite the risk, I offer this work. My close friend and mentor Joe Fletcher has posed a very demanding mandate. "Tell us what you believe and why and what that has to do with medicine." I believe the time has come for me to move beyond mimicking, reporting, and restating the work of others and at last present something of my own sweat and tears, a fragment from an accumulation of life experiences, something living and fresh.

This work represents the collected log of my own journey. When our children are asked what their dad does for a living, they stumble in explanation, "He is a doctor—a minister—he teaches ethics in a medical school—I'm not really sure what he does!" Actually, twenty years of adventuring in this new profession called bioethics have not afforded their father much greater clarity. The privilege of reflecting philosophically and theologically about science, technology, and medical practice, though fashionable and even faddish as a profession, is still an ill-defined and obscure art. In this

book I invite you to join me in a tough but fascinating intellectual
struggle—one made necessary by the practical decisions of birth
and death which we must now all face.

INTRODUCTION

This forms the first part of a major work which will attempt to
present a comprehensive theology of bioscience and health care for
the end of this millennium. This endeavor might be called *Religio
Medici 2000* after Thomas Browne's classic work. This particular
book on birth, as well as its sequel on death, is the outcropping of
two decades of clinical learning, listening, teaching, and sharing the
struggle with people as they make and live with their decisions.

It is a book about ethics. Ethics is the discipline which thinks
about what we should value and how we should behave. It is not
the science of how we value and behave; that is the domain of so-
ciology and behavioral science. It is not the science of how we have
valued and behaved; that is the domain of history. Ethics ponders
how we ought now to value and behave.

The reader will find this book as much a new proposal for ethical theoretics as one of perinatal pragmatics. Though it presents
analyses and persuasions about the great birth questions of abortion, surrogacy, infanticide, amniocentesis, population, genetics,
and others, it will take these much-discussed questions as vehicles
by which to propose a new way of looking at ethics. I believe the
reader will find here a comprehensive ethic that will consider various dimensions of the personal and collective moral capacity: natural, rational, political, and theological. Using Charles Hartshorne's
image, it will attempt to balance extreme temporalism and extreme
eternalism (dangers in philosophy and ethics) by arching a rainbow
of colors between those two pots of gold. It will look at the faculties
of the "moral soul" and the aspects of reality to which they correspond. Ethics is "being true" to ourselves and to the Transcendent.
Some sense of *humanum* and *divinum*—accession to that which is
penultimate and ultimate—forms the basis of all ethics.

Why is this more complicated ethic required? Simply because
the age-old work of understanding and transforming the human being has reached an intense pitch in our time. This feverish scientific
and technological project of the last two centuries can be searched
out and evaluated by exploring the transformations of the thresholds of birth and death. These thresholds will be explored in order

to hold together experiences and challenges that inevitably affect each other. Birth and death are inextricably intertwined one with the other. Interventions at the birth threshold influence what will happen and what we must do at the threshold of death. The "population explosion," for example, is caused as much by diminished death rate as it is by increased birth rate.

I start with genesis, with beginnings. Not only does this make chronological sense, but it acknowledges the concentrated moral fascination that has always been drawn to sexuality, birth, and related issues. Those who trouble themselves with medical philosophy find themselves absorbed with questions of sexual, genetic, and pediatric ethics.

NATIVITY AND NATALITY

The ethical standpoint which will be taken in this volume on birth calls into question a prevalent position by reaffirming a traditional one. The current dominant birth ethic, which can be called one of rational technique, is a natality ethic somewhat discordant with our normative nativity tradition. Every age thinks, values, and operates in terms of a dominant ethos. The current ideology of birth, which emphasizes objectivity, manipulability, and interchangeability, stands in stark contrast to the classical theistic and humanistic vision. This latter way of considering and doing things was one of mystical intersubjectivity and pathetic cohumanity. We have moved from an ethic of grateful acceptance and mutual support with whatever life gave us to one where we writhe in anger and impute blame when everything is not perfect. In the traditional ethic we are born from and die into the love of God. In the new pragmatic ethic all good consists in sheer human will, power, and control. The older humanistic perspective needs to be restored to save us from a wide range of degradations.

Today's mythos is exemplified by Baby Fae, the child in California whose damaged heart was removed shortly after birth and replaced by a baboon's heart. We now look scientifically and technically at cells, tissues, and organs with a view to fixing or replacing the parts which malfunction. Consider the little child in Chicago who undergoes four liver transplants or the baby in California who receives the heart of an anencephalic baby born in Canada or a little girl in Pittsburgh who receives a modified carriage transplant of liver, intestines, and the rest. All these cases symbolize both the glory and sadness of a novel moral situation arising among us as a new mentality about parents, conception, birth, and child life comes to characterize late twentieth-century America. The same revolution is found in other cultures where the Western scientific worldview and technology have displaced traditional beliefs and values. We are left in a bewildering situation because our deeper traditional convictions conflict with the values inherent in current technological capacities.

Throughout this volume the thesis unfolds that our present scientific perspectives toward mother and child must not be abandoned but must be augmented by knowledge and practice that move beyond the rational and technical. The glory of present powers need not be annulled but should be deepened by rejoining them to perennial wisdom. Just as we know our eyes can see only a part of the color spectrum and our ears hear only a part of the sound spectrum, so we must learn to lay open our moral perception to deeper and higher colors, tones, and signals. We must temper our mania to manipulate life infinitely, borne of our perpetual dissatisfaction with what is and our desire to fashion something different. A multicolored spectrum of moral colors, a multichanneled symphony of moral sounds, can enlarge our ethical consciousness. Life situations, agonizing choices about birth and babies, open up dimensions of a moral universe of meanings which resonate with cognate capacities, some latent or dormant, in our moral souls. This book calls on us to open up all channels and put on moral infrared and ultraviolet viewers so that we can more adequately see the birth spectacle before us and respond with greater resonance to the moral symphony of the universe.

TRANSIT TO NATALITY

We can now begin our journey together. In this phase of the journey we will follow the course of concerns that mark conception, birth, infancy, and childhood. The reader is invited to consider a succession of subjects in the light of a progression of principles. Each component of an ethical theory will be elaborated in conjunction with a particular perinatal question. Please do not view this arrangement as making artificial pigeonholes. I want merely to suggest a richer repertoire of value which can help us in all the decisions of life. I pick particular perinatal problems to illustrate given parameters of ethics because of their special pertinence to that ethical idea and not to rule out the others.

We will begin by reconsidering the problem of human pro-creation and population expansion, accenting the dimensions of ecological ethics. Along the way we will pass other signposts: apoc-alyptic, biologic, psychic, philosophical, epistemic, historical, polit-ical, theological, and eschatological. In a summary synthesis, we will weave these all together into one fabric of ethics. For now, they will be used as windows through which to view a spectrum of na-tality issues, from AIDS to the care of young children. There is an interplay among all of these questions. For example, genetic diagno-sis, abortion, and postnatal care of impoverished children must be viewed synoptically and synthetically. They relate to each other and affect each other. There is also a wider interplay, which is the reason this volume will have a sequel dealing with mortality. Birth and death intertwine not only in the sheer fact that the rates of each must find some semblance of equilibrium but also as they partici-pate together in the universal drama of suffering and in the meaning and mystery of life.

As Homer sings in the *Iliad:* "As is the generation of leaves, so is that of humanity. The wind scatters the leaves on the ground, but the live timber burgeons with leaves again in the season of spring returning. So one generation of men will grow while another dies."[1] We begin with reflections about that generation which is coming into being and growing.

1 Ecological Ethics of Heaven and Earth:

POPULATION EXPANSION

Respect of natural resources of our planet must be part of everyone's conscience. Each man must avoid actions which can damage purity of environment.

Pope John Paul II, "Mass on Dolomite Alps in Northern Italy," July 12, 1987

The 1980 *Global 2000 Report to the President* states the ecological problem in its stark reality, citing a "potential for global problems of alarming proportions."

Environmental, resource, and population stresses are intensifying and will increasingly determine the quality of human life on our planet. These stresses are already severe enough to deny millions of people basic needs for food, shelter, health and jobs, or any hope for betterment. At the same time, the earth's carrying capacity—the ability of biological systems to provide re-

1

> sources for human needs—is eroding. The trends . . . suggest
> strongly a progressive degradation and impoverishment of the
> earth's natural resources base.[1]

The report proceeds to describe a world where population rapidly expands while resources to sustain quality life rapidly contract. The detailed documentation of threat to the life-giving resources of food, fisheries, forests, water, and energy is juxtaposed against the drama of more and more people with less and less facility to survive, let alone live well in an increasingly harsh and improvident world.

Population expansion is held to be one of the continuing factors in this scenario of desperation. The world's population will grow from 4 billion in 1975 to 6.35 billion in 2000. Fully 90 percent of the growth will occur in the poorest countries. The crisis is compounded by the possibility of zero growth, perhaps depopulation, in the developed world.[2] For much of the poor of the globe, the annual GNP per capita is expected to remain below two hundred dollars. Arable land resources are barely remaining stable, which means that food prices will increase, while ability to provide self-sustenance will weaken.

Immediately the crisis takes on the character of ethical pathos, the sublime admixture of suffering and saving which we will contend is the crux of morality. The dialectic of need evoking help is evident. When reports from the Club of Rome and Global 2000 counsel "Cease multiplying or beware" and when a *New York Times* book review of *The Birth Dearth* is entitled "Be Fruitful or Be Sorry,"[3] we see quickly the ethical dynamics of population expansion. Power and resources build up in some sectors, need and impoverishment intensify in others. An ethics of justice and sacrifice, therefore, becomes increasingly necessary for the survival of both sectors.

By 2030 the world's population will reach 10 billion, and 30 billion by the end of the twenty-first century. We now see the practical necessity of an ethic that has ecological, apocalyptic, and eschatological tenor along with the more customary features of morality. We are dealing with cataclysm in Nature and in history. Nero could fiddle while Rome burned, and Louis Catorce could condemn the future to the flood, but if we forsake the future, it will indeed be damned. The crisis of population serves to illustrate the ecological feature of a comprehensive ethic. The world which cradles our life is being pushed to the limits of its providence. "Extinctions of plant and animal species will increase dramatically. Hundreds of thousands of species—perhaps as many as 20 percent of all species on earth—will be irretrievably lost as their habitats vanish, especially in tropical forests."[4] As we near the end of this millennium, 25 percent of the world's population will need wood fuel for heat and cooking, while the usable stands of forest will be diminished by 50 percent. A world to which we have been called in conscience as stewards, to be fruitful, to fill, to replenish, now threatens to degrade and disintegrate before us. What is the nature of the crisis and a fitting moral response?

THE POPULATION CRISIS

Population projections are based on a complex equation which includes five factors: crude birthrate, crude death rate, growth rate (birth/death differential and migration), rate of natural increase, and total fertility rate. Population projections based on these indices are visualized on figures 1 and 2.[5]

The graphics make clear these developments. First, world population is growing dramatically as a result of increasing birthrates and decreasing death rates. Second, the building of population is concentrated in the less-developed world, with a proportionate decrease in the developed world. (This might be a salutary development. A teacher from India once remarked that one American child was the equivalent of twenty-five of his in terms of the resources consumed during a lifetime.) Third, in the less-developed world the great majority of population increase will be in infants and children. In the developed world the high increase will come in the elderly, especially women.

Every country in the world has some formal or informal family-planning activity. Programs range from those completely voluntary with widespread availability of contraception and sterilization (Canada) to state-induced policies with highly suggestive, even mandatory, sanctions (China). Although China's new eugenics measures have dramatically changed doomsday predictions on the mainland, elsewhere in Asia (India, Indonesia, Bangladesh, and Pakistan), Africa (in nations like Egypt and Nigeria), and Latin American (in nations like Mexico), the projections are still frightening. In the United States, dramatic growth is projected among the black, hispanic, and Asian populations, with immigration enhancing the numbers.

What analysis and interpretation should be brought to these data from the ethical point of view? By some twist of history the wealth and well-being of the part of the world that has experienced rapid economic growth since the early Modern Age and the Indus-

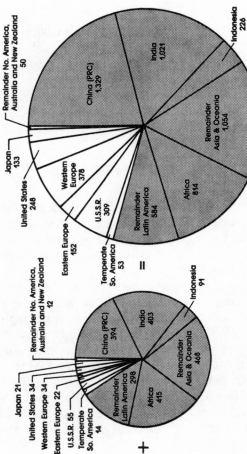

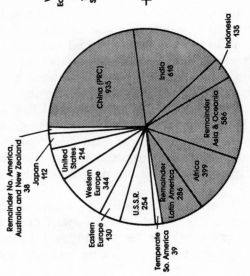

Figure 2-1. Twenty-five years of world population growth, medium series.

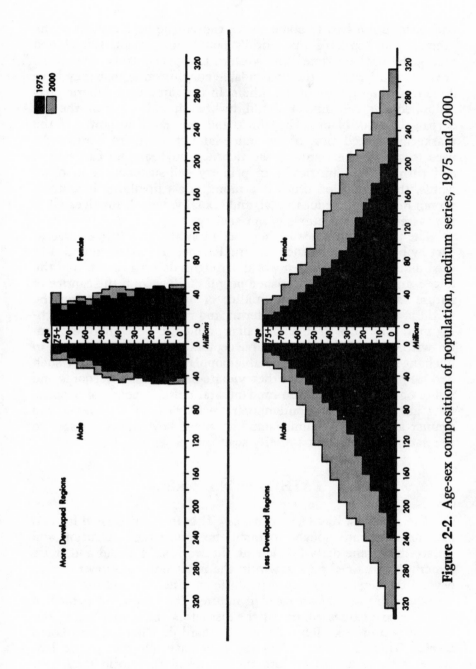

Figure 2-2. Age-sex composition of population, medium series, 1975 and 2000.

trial Revolution has, in some sense, caused the depreciation of the other. If one-tenth of the world's population (Japan, the United States, the Arab oil states, and western Europe) controls nine-tenths of the world's wealth, the unavoidable conclusion is that they have done it at the expense of the others. In the same way, America has fashioned, and continues to build, its wealth and power on the underpaid labor of blacks, Hispanics, and women. The power of the market has forced more of the arable land of the Third World to be used to satiate the wants of the rich (e.g. soybeans for cattle feed) and turn those countries from primary self-sustenance. In other words, the population crisis is a moral crisis involving industrial, economic, housing, educational, and sexual values. It involves all of the systems and structures of our society.

The population crisis is therefore a moral crisis. It is created in part by human malevolence and indifference. It is also grounded in the brokenness of the fallen world. Drought, desertification, and the forced migration of impoverished peoples follow from the caprice of nature as much as from the malice of human beings. When the world is viewed in terms of suffering and redemption, our overarching moral response to this particular problem is an equipoise of anger with demand for change and acceptance of the pain inherent in unchangeable tragedies. Acceptable population policies reflect such natural prudence, but when they violate basic human freedoms and rights or abrogate the more fundamental cultural goods of peoples, they are ill advised. Contemporary ecological ethics take shape against a backdrop of understanding about how humans relate to the natural world. Let us briefly scan this background.

PATHOS IN NATURE

The ancients, like Heraclitus, saw flux in nature. Then for two millennia humans sought to tame the tempestuous creation and satisfy the serene deity by viewing the world as a placid and static system. It remained for Darwin in the nineteenth century to move beyond the serene confidence in static specific forms of life and re-introduce the idea of struggle in nature. The quality of pathos in nature is best expressed, not by the dissectors and reductionists, but by lyric writers like René Dubos, Teilhard de Chardin, and Loren Eiseley. Though all are scientists, they have felt that poetic language is necessary to capture the nature of the world they have come to know.

For Dubos, for example, it is the presence of disease and healing and the miracle of adaptation which enables nature to repair the damage of breakage and accident that constitutes the redemptive mystery of creation. "The ability to evolve is ... an essential attribute of life. ... These changes progressively result in the production of new forms of life. ... Diversity accounts in large part for the self-repairing processes which tend to occur spontaneously when accidents disturb the natural order of things—hence the adaptability and resilience of the living earth. It accounts also for the adaptability, resilience, and richness of human life."[6] If nature itself exhibits certain patterns of pathos and regeneration, then a cosmic or ecological ethic will seek out a delicate balance of dominance and resonance, subjugation and resignation, offsetting where possible the deleterious effect of the damaging processes on humans, but otherwise attempting to harmonize human action with the movements, rhythms, and causalities of nature.

A good example of this delicate kind of management would be the control we seek over the microbial world. In countering infection generally, in antibiotic prophylaxis present in vaccines and biologicals, even in the extreme case of controlling exposure in immunosuppressed or immunodeficient persons (e.g. SCID, or Severe Combined Immunological Deficiency, patients), a balance of attack and acceptance is necessary. We accept a certain microbial flora as healthy. The bugs in our intestines are welcome and indeed life-saving inhabitants. It is the outrageous inhabitation that must be checked. In medical therapy as well as in ethics more generally, transformative values such as amelioration, improvement, and justice will always interplay with resignative values such as care, consolation, and serenity. By this light let us critically evaluate some of the population proposals that have been put forward.

PROPOSALS OF POPULATION ETHICS

Four representative moral policies for population management range from the overly aggressive to the overly acquiescent, with two moderate options in between. To survey other approaches will allow us to position the perspective generated by the ethical system we are proposing. It will also allow us, by way of critical comment, to set the stage for a discussion of an ecological ethic that is enriched by the other components under review.

Overly aggressive scenarios of population control exist in uto-

pian literature and in limited utopian experiments. The *Republic* of
Plato, the *Utopia* of Thomas More, and Huxley's *Brave New World*
are examples of ideal states where not only is population kept under
control in numbers and quality, but birth is positively engineered to
yield the desired human power and the variegation of social skills
required. Though the Shakers' eschatological sexual policies extinguish population altogether, the central motivation in such utopian
sectors is usually not population management per se.

In the early decades of the twentieth century, we saw the first
examples of forceful policies of population management. Throughout Europe, America, and Great Britain, sweeping designs and
actual programs for contraception and family planning were introduced. Though governmental intervention and grand schemes of eugenic sterilization were envisioned by some, most efforts were
educational activities, door-to-door appeals among the grass-roots
population. The desire to provide information and "appliances" for
families sought to intercept the necessity of intercourse leading to
pregnancy. Margaret Sanger's pamphlet *Family Limitation*, written
in 1914 at the threshold of the Great War, glimpsed calamity in the
offing. Crisis was impending because of the excess fertility of the
poor in a time of economic hardship. Speaking of the Rivertown
where she herself was born the sixth of eleven children to a tuber-
cular mother, she wrote:

> Along the river flats lived the factory workers, chiefly Irish; on
> the heights above the rolling clouds of smoke that belched from
> the chimneys lived the owners and executives. The tiny gardens
> of the former were asprawl with children; in the gardens on the
> hills only two or three played. This contrast made a track in my
> mind: large families were associated with poverty, toil, unem-
> ployment, drunkenness, cruelty, fighting, jails; the small ones
> with cleanliness, leisure, freedom, light, space, sunshine.[7]

The general mood of the times expressed the belief that excessive
propagation endangered both the poor families themselves and the
larger society that was obliged to provide welfare.

In New York City, the journal *Medical Review of Reviews* hired
several down-and-outers to walk among the crowded districts of the
city with placards which read:

> I am a burden to myself and the state.
> Should I be allowed to propagate?

I have no opportunity to educate or feed my children.
They may become criminals.
Would the prisons and asylums be filled
if my kind had no children?
I cannot read this sign.
By what right have I children?[8]

These ideas now seem obscurantist and offensive. But they were once widely held. When the national socialists came to power in Germany in the 1930s and started to talk about "excess mouths to feed" and the burden of "worthless lives" on the state, they were drawing many of their ideas from earlier American materials. Programs of that era were harsh not only in their ideology and propaganda but also in the way they reflected and created a public mood of contempt for the poor.

Germaine Greer concludes that this period accomplished very little in the way of securing power and reproductive freedom for women or of establishing stability. "What they did do was create the precedent for the invasion of privacy which made reproductive behavior a public matter and placed its regulation in the hands of the medical and pharmaceutical [and we might add the political] establishment."[9] The intensely alarmist visions of population explosion and the condemnation-laden programs to avert disaster that marked the early twentieth century exaggerated a suffering pathos in society and an excessive optimism about ameliorative strategies. This distorted reading of pathos yielded a distorted ethos. The ethic was too little filled with compassion and sympathy. The desire was to do away with problems rather than understand and share people's difficulties and actually help them. While disguised as an ethic of fellow feeling, it was actually a desire to be rid of a problem, an apathetic desire for noninvolvement.

Moderately aggressive programs of population control, set in motion in the 1960s, represent a second approach to population management. In the 1967 provisions of the Social Security Act, the stipulates on aid to families with dependent children were altered (1) to require that at least 6 percent of all funds available for maternal and child care be earmarked for family planning, and (2) to direct all the states to offer family-planning services to present, past, and potential AFDC recipients in an effort to reduce illegitimate births and lower welfare expenses.[10] This was the era of public and quasipublic family-planning agencies. Public sentiment to "do something" about the population crisis was fueled by the reports of

University of Chicago sociologist Philip Hauser, who, though himself a man of exceptional moral vision, gave credence to bigoted
views that the black population was growing at frightful rates.

In the late 1960s many branches of government came to support programs of population control. As Thomas Littlewood observed, "Bills were introduced in many state legislatures proposing
mandatory sterilization after a specified number of illegitimate
pregnancies."[11] It was at about this time that courses in medical
ethics began to appear in the medical centers of the United States.
The initial issue that captured our attention was the choosing of
recipients for the few available kidneys and then hearts for transplantation. We also thought and wrote about the appropriateness of
withdrawing life-sustaining treatment and of sickness-induced suicide. Strangely, the issue of encouraged, if not coerced, sterilization
of poor mothers in the charity hospitals of the land did not become
a major issue. I can remember such procedures being routinely performed at the county hospital where I worked. (The woman who
headed up the program was something of a folk hero.) At that time
sterilization was construed, even by woman's advocacy groups, as
giving women greater freedom over their own bodies. Only when
the feminist movement shifted its concern and looked at the im-
plicit violation of women did this attitude change.

At the same time, the global concerns of population expansion
were also growing. Various governments in the developing lands
sought to implement programs with aid from the developed countries and from great private foundations. These programs were
somewhat more salutary in effect, since they did not conceal fear
and contempt regarding the receivers, nor did they hold out the
prospect of economic benefit to the dispensers.

Generally considered, the moderate programs taught us important lessons about human freedom in moral choice—that, while the
scientific, educational, and political efforts to constrain rapid population growth were well founded, they had to be offered when the
persons concerned needed and wanted them and not when they
served some ulterior expedient. At this point, moral reflection on
population ethics began to profit from ecological (resource exhaus-
tion), historical (Nazi eugenics), political (what government can appropriately do), and other vectors of ethics. The main ethical insight
came when planners became more careful of drawing a calculus of
suffering, checking more carefully not to project their own comforts
onto the sufferings of others.

The moral inadequacy of highly managed and moderately aggressive programs lies in their narrow utilitarian focus. Narrow numerical calculations are made to determine how many bodies are needed and how many mouths can be fed. While this might make sense in computational logic, it makes little sense with other focal points on our moral continuum. For all we know, the goods of a local or global society might better be served against some future contingency by multitudes rather than carefully preplanned allotments—for instance, if population were decimated by a nuclear disaster or a pandemic.

A second critical question concerns whether the policies acknowledge the mystery and dignity of human persons. Judaism for the most part is a pronatal tradition. One of the reasons this people has sustained such an ethical heritage long after agricultural people needed farmhands and old-age security is the messianic notion that, one day somewhere, one will be born who will enrich and save the human family. Therefore each life is a divine gift and as such is precious and inviolable. This redemptive note—the correlate of our suffering axis of ethics—casts a different light on most choices.

Third, a *moderately resigned* ecological ethic of population growth has been achieved in modern Japan. This moral posture is rooted in the general deference, respect, and civility of the Japanese people. Acutely aware of the geographical constraints imposed by the archipelago, chastened into acceptance of natural limitations by foolhardy expansionist policies of the past, the country has moved beyond the saddening infanticide and abortion measures of recent history to a more wholesome, equilibrium-maintaining practice of population control. The secret seems to be the condom. Undergirded by a social psychology of gentle encouragement, "love boxes" are deposited with families by health workers or passed from neighbor to neighbor. The boxes contain supplies for six months, which on return visit are paid for and replenished; 80 percent of Japanese couples use the male prophylactics.

A very unique and exemplary philosophy of suffering and ecological ethic is found on these islands, which support 120 million people, one consonant with a people who invented the rock garden and who produced Kazoh Kitamori, author of *Theology of the Pain of God.*[12] How have the Japanese dealt with the pain of God and the pain of life that is the inevitable concomitant of transferring life to a new generation or denying that transfer?

Historically, Japan dealt with the pain of birth by dramatic measures. The *mabiki* policy of the late nineteenth and early twentieth century ensured that the human crop was "thinned out" by infanticide. The ancient ritual of Hinoeuma, the year of the horse, in which no children were to be born, still had effect as late as 1966. Dr. Ogino's ovulation cycle abstinence program gained worldwide interest. Widespread abortion gained acceptance after the war, as did the penitent visits to the temples of Jizo to pray for the souls of the unborn children. Those who have studied the Japanese population phenomenon have noted great attention paid to the suffering placed on women in the entire burden of conception and pregnancy. In a society so filled with grace and gentleness, we might expect this accent to deal with the repressed violence of spirit.[13]

Our ethical perspective looks favorably on the Japanese experience because of its thoughtful concern with an ecological ethic and its sensitivity to the agonal aspects of procreation. It is no surprise that modern Japan has at some points surpassed the United States as the economic leader of the world. Their careful ecological and economic ethos (concerned with house/management, or *oikos*), has brought this kind of success, even though it has been at the cost of trade surpluses that have harmed other countries. The concern for house sustenance, when extended to the whole *oikoumenē*—the whole inhabited world—could someday bring abundant and satisfying life to the people of the whole world. But this eschatological vision must wait to be elaborated later.

In a comprehensive pathetic ethic such as we will elaborate, with dimensions ranging from the ecological to the eschatological, pleasure in life is concomitant with the sensitive bearing and sharing of pain. This is one of the essential teachings of ethics in the great traditions and is the cornerstone of our system. The presence of suffering—in poverty, in infant mortality, in denied opportunity to youth—is rampant in our world. Yet thanks to (largely Japanese) electronics, the world's pain is daily brought before our very eyes. It remains to be seen whether this unprecedented cognizance—instantaneous and intense—will prompt us to greater action or to greater apathy. The first signs are not good. In the present political atmosphere of the West, we cannot bear or do not care to see suffering. We turn off the TV sets or turn to bromide programs. But if we do receive it, share it, and seek where possible to relieve it, we may know again the contentment of acts well done, lives well lived.

There is yet another ethical approach to the population crisis which sits very close to the ethical paradigm we are proposing but is not without its drawbacks. The moral teaching of the Roman Catholic church expressed in *Humanae Vitae* (1968) and the "Instruction on Birth Science" (1987) sets forth a doctrine which, though exemplary and preserving deep values, is *overly resigned* to the problems at hand.

Humanae Vitae is based on three central premises. First, a central vocation of human beings—indeed, a reason for their being—is to propagate and educate children. Second, the unitive and procreative dimensions of human nature must not be severed. Sexuality must always remain open, if possible, to the transmission of life. Finally, any interruption of the generative process, whether abortion, sterilization, or contraception, is proscribed.[14]

The "Instruction on Respect for Human Life in Its Origins and on the Dignity of Procreation" (1987) extended the same general principles to new questions such as surrogacy and in-vitro fertilization. This latter document picks up better than any modern text the extreme irony of procreation that reveals the moral bewilderment of the modern world at the point of this power and responsibility. What has happened to the human family when some persons, say the 20 percent organically infertile or the 70 percent of American women who for various reasons are infertile, are so desperate to have a child that they will go to the extraordinary measures of IVF, surrogacy, or an expensive Korean purchase to have a baby, while at the same time, other countless persons are equally desperate to ensure that they do not have a child and resort to abortion?[15]

The genius of the Catholic document is that it sees what is happening morally in this strange contradiction, that some vicariously suffer for the many. One of the phenomena of pain sharing and pain bearing in our world is that suffering is often concentrated in the few or the one. The concentration of burden bearing (a metaphor of load carrying and pregnancy) was placed in the Jew Jesus as his body weight and the sin of the world was suspended on the spikes, pounded into the Golgotha tree. That vicarious act at the turning point of history and the call for discipleship from within that image to "bear ye one another's burdens" (Gal. 6:2) are vivid examples of the way in which the weight of suffering is either concentrated or distributed. The messianic history of the Jews, if fathomable in any way, may be understood as their vicarious bearing of the sin of the world for its redemption. The unborn who never see the light bear in some secret way the suffering of the world. Today AIDS victims and the elderly poor also bear a vicarious suffering for a world gone wrong.

The weakness of Roman Catholic teaching on population ethics is a cruciform theology that is too stoic. While the system of value is not completely masochistic in its willingness to abide the suffering its persuasion on contraception creates, it comes close. It is an ethic that is so resigned to natural inevitability that it fails to celebrate sufficiently the scientific and technological genius—indeed, the providential grace—of birth science.[16] In a lecture on the Instruction at the University of Chicago, Cardinal Bernadin quoted with favor this passage from one of my essays: "The Instruction affirms a much-threatened normative value of the natural goodness and sacred mystery of birth. Regrettably, in its desire to preserve the deeply human nature of procreation, it plays down the salutary potential of science to ameliorate incapacity in the same procreative gift."[17] Redemptive power is released into the world in the desire we have to alleviate suffering and provide health for one another. Science and technology are aspects of this power.

The Roman Catholic view also overaccents the apocalyptic and eschatological aspects of ethics in its acclaim of celibacy and the implied moral inferiority of the marriage state. Drawn from the recesses of primitive Christian history, where the imminent end of time and the return of Christ was expected, an ascetic ideal prompted that community along with the Dead Sea Essenes and other communities to refrain from marriage and procreation. As a result, a strain of disparagement of the body and human sexuality entered Christian teaching which can be found in thinkers from Augustine to Pope John Paul II. Though the teaching accepts one component of a creative and comprehensive ethic, it contradicts the body-affirmation doctrine even of its own biblical tradition. This spiritualization also causes the Roman Catholic tradition, like some Holiness traditions of Israel, to be overly fascinated with the techniques of sexuality to the neglect of deeper meanings and outcomes. The interest in coitus interruptus, like onanism, diverts attention from sexuality as a natural and desirable good.

The great contribution of the Roman tradition has been its Christocentric theology and ethic of natality. More than any other tradition or way of life in the modern world, this heritage reminds the world of the brokenness at the center of creation, of redemptive, sacrificial love that has gone to the heart of the matter, and of the imperative to identify with need and reconcile suffering so that pain is transfigured into pleasure and death into life. This is the focus of an ecological ethic that emerges in the moral system we are setting forth.

AN ECOLOGICAL ETHIC

Paul Ehrlich, professor of biological and population studies at Stanford, the scientist who first reminded us of the population bomb, has argued that a transformation of ecological ethics and a deemphasized people ethic is the best hope for survival of life on earth.

> The main hope for changing humanity's present course may lie less with politics . . . than in the development of a world view drawn partly from ecological principles—in the so-called deep ecology movement. . . . Most of its adherents favor a much less anthropocentric, more egalitarian world, with greater emphasis on empathy and less on scientific rationality. . . . I am convinced that such a quasi-religious movement, one concerned with the need to change the values that now govern much of human activity, is essential to the persistence of our civilization.[18]

A reverential ethic has more to do with people than nature, yet Ehrlich makes a forceful point. We have begun to give shape to the ecological component of an ethic of suffering, death, and transfiguration. We have offered comments to several representative proposals of population ethics. These comments have served to suggest what the ethic we are sketching would offer by way of guiding values to the population crisis. In order to elaborate that ecological ethic further, let us look now at two moral features which arise when we conceive of our environment as habitat, an ecological and economic living place. As noted, the Greek word *oikos*, the root word of *ecology* and *economy*, conveys the idea that we share an abode, an abiding place. Here we share, suffer, and flourish together. In this ecumenical habitat the weight of need and suffering is either absorbed by mutual provision and sacrifice and thereby transformed into life and morale (resurrection, or the spirit of renewal), or it deteriorates into hoarding, overuse, violence, and ultimately degradation and damnation.

One of the most perceptive essays of our time, Garrett Hardin's *The Tragedy of the Commons*, calls our attention to the ethical distortion of cornering the market, of establishing the turf, excluding interlopers, and exhausting the habitat so as to avoid pain, sacrifice, and generosity.[19] This now-classic text draws as a centerpiece a passage from Whitehead which speaks of the tragicomic central act around which the grand drama of life is acted out. The script of this hinge story is very close to the play within the play that we are placing at the center stage of our moral system. Whitehead wrote: "The essence of dramatic tragedy is not unhappiness. It resides in the solemnity of the remorseless working of things."

"Ye shall have a song," wrote Randall Thompson in his hymn *The Peaceable Kingdom*, "as in the night when a holy solemnity is kept." The span and horizons of our existence and the givenness of our cosmos is the sacrament, the song, the harmony amid the cacophony of life. Within boundaries we come to know the mystery of our personal and communal being. In coming to terms with the inevitable contours of our freedom and the ambit of our habitat, we are released to the stewardship and service which is authentic freedom.

Hardin draws several moral inferences from this idea of tragedy, which are also the imperatives that our ethic of suffering and succor yields. First, we must not continue to long for or rely on technical solutions to the traumas of population and ecology. A crisis by its very nature invites ethical, not technical, response. Rather than leave one's comfortable apathy and risk sympathy, rather than forgo immediate enjoyment and venture the frugality of the gift *simplicitas*, we concoct ever more imaginative technical fixes. Each fix eventually requires a counterfix. In response to the population challenge, we will colonize outer space, farm the seas, recombine DNA, and fashion oil-spill-eating bacteria, we say. Only one problem—who will eat the oil-eaters? What do we do with the wreckage of the last technological fix—the last Andromeda strain?

A closely related moral position that Hardin critiques is the view that things will take care of themselves. Adam Smith's "hidden hand" doctrine is molded by the theologian-economist's misreading of Calvin's doctrine of providence. When combined with a Darwinian ethic, this erroneous view believes that adaptation will inevitably occur. The fertility of the bell-jar fruit-fly population will diminish, nongenerative homosexuality will increase, as will violence, so that the crowding will eventually check the acceleration of population. Another aspect of the "hidden hand" doctrine holds that self-interest—for example, unrestrained procreation—is ultimately productive of social good. The individual who "intends only his own gain" is, as it were, led by an invisible hand to promote "the public interest." The modern economic version of this myth is the trickle-down theory of economics, which believes that, when wealth is built up to overflowing in some places, it will spill over to the benefit of those all around. The trouble with the idea is twofold: first, the accumulation of wealth and power in one sector depends in part on relinquishment or turnover from other sectors. Second, the trickle-down effect theory results in just trickles—and such droppings serve only to increase dependence and rage.

A slight critique that our moral approach would offer to Hardin's version of ecological ethics comes at the point of whether or not we live in a finite world. If the world is closed and finite, the kind of exquisite give-and-take that Hardin splendidly commends is mandatory. This book would argue that the posture of ecological awe and social justice that he commends is absolutely obligatory, not because we live in a closed system but because the sacrifice at the heart of reality grounds our authentic humanness in that same posture. Morally fulfilled existence is that which takes gently and gives generously. Second, serendipity based on justice and generosity yields new possibilities. Calvin's doctrine of providence in the ecosphere (ecology and economics) is based on the manna doctrine of Scripture (Exodus 16; 2 Corinthians 8), whereby faithful stewardship and concern for the other brings forth more than appears to be available—a *more* sufficient for every need.

The central section of Hardin's essay rehearses the old metaphor of the commons. The cattle graze on the common village green. Each farmer knows the exact number from his herd that can graze along with the same number of head from his colleague's herd. The tragedy is triggered when in freedom we all seek to maximize our own interest. This inevitably leads each person to sneak one more animal onto the green when we think no one is watching, until the carrying capacity of the commons eventually collapses and everyone goes down together as the dry grass blows away in the wind.

While greed, acquisition, and exploitation have become an ingrained pattern, Hardin shows how nature itself commends to us the approach of "psychological denial" as being more advantageous even in terms of "natural selection." This ascetic, frugal pattern of ecological ethics, reminiscent of Benedictine and Franciscan stewardship, embodies a reverence for nature and conforms with an ethic of cosmic sensibility. In a recent study of Aristotle's doctrine of moderation, Charles Hartshorne writes in the same mood. "Starvation is not good, overeating is not good. . . . Well did Aristotle say that virtues in contrast to vices are judicious means between contrary extremes."[20] Overpowering and overreaching inevitably weakens and diminishes its agent and the field of life.

Aristotle, the Greeks, and many ancient peoples of western Asia had a perspective on tragedy that, though different from the Semitic vision, had the same effect. *Hubris* was the human desire to overcome limitations, to fail to accept the place and purpose that was structured into one's being and into the natural world. When enriched by the Hebrew-Christian doctrine of creation and fall, we have here a helpful sense of the evil and good prospect that stands before us. For the Jew, humankind is fallen (though perhaps not along with the whole natural creation as in Christianity). Humans are also capable, indeed prone, to misdirect freedom to the harm and destruction of self, others, and our world. In both Hellenic and Hebraic views of the fall (primal tragedy) and perpetual temptation, humans, very much as in Hardin's image, find it impossible not to go too far. In Christian speech, *non posse non peccare* (it is not possible not to go wrong).

But, we must ask, if the cosmos and the human family are a divine creation, why are we locked into such a tragedy? Why is human freedom invariably misdirected? Why is it impossible not to sin? Here we come to the heartland of the metaphysics and meta-ethics. Where suffering, death, and transfiguration constitute the basic paradigm of reality and therefore the pattern of good/evil and ethics, the tragedy of the creation becomes the clue to its transfiguration. The sin of humankind is the secret of its salvation. Sickness is the key to health, death to life. What has gone wrong in the world (not what is wrong or just what is) portrays for us what was meant to be and what could be. In cosmic or ecological ethics, therefore, we are not given to romantic idolization, cynical depreciation, or discouraged resignation about the world. We are rather encouraged to make commitments to honor, safe-keep, and build the earth. We are to help the world along, as Chauncy Gardner did in the film *Being There*, nudging it in directions of its potential and providence. In words that Hardin's thoughtful essay suggests, creation doctrines offer us a commons, a garden, a place set aside for our intending, tending, and stewardship.

A second strand of ecological ethics emphasizes economics. Population concerns always intertwine with the concerns of poverty. If indeed we can speak of synergy and creative potential within the constraints of nature, it will be found in imaginative resource utilization and economic management. Although we cannot affirm the hidden-hand or trickle-down theory of economics, we do affirm the possibility of making the most of the resources at hand, keeping them working in generosity and justice for the benefit of all.

We have argued that an ethics fit for the world we live in and relevant to the problems we face begins with a cosmic or ecological dimension. The basic principle of our system—suffering, death, and transfiguration—serves as a leitmotif, drawing together concerns of stewardship of the natural world; euthenics, or the improvement of human environment; and attention to human needs and to the particular concerns of the population crisis. What attitudinal response and action does this ethic call forth? Suffering, sacrifice, and stewardship have emerged as prominent features of an ecological ethic. There will be pain, persistent crisis, and imperfection in nature, since the world is fallen and through cosmic agony is becoming new. We will not find utopia, nor should we demand it through escape into sedated nonworlds. Rather, we should share what we have received as if it were a gift and not a possession, a gift given to use for the purpose of enlarging it through expenditure. Among the committed, sacrifice is a joyous act, enriching the giver.

Finally, our ethic calls for an enduring commitment to tend the garden of this earth. We are to husband its growth, transport its providence, and replenish it for new growth. This pattern of responsibility—sacrifice, expenditure, and renewal—is the ethical resonance to the redemptive throb we find at the heart of reality. To conclude this chapter on population ethics, let us now appropriate the moral ideas we have sketched to the real world in which we find ourselves and to the concerns before us just now. Let us consider the global and the provincial case.

The global crisis is before us. World population is now at 5 billion and certainly moving toward 10 billion. At that level experts feel there is some chance of leveling off. Some Asian, African, and Latin American countries (Kenya, for example) are growing at a precipitous rate, already threatening resources. The challenge at the international level is to see if national planning and mutual assistance can gain control before nature solves the problem for us. If we cannot bring orderly equilibrium and maintenance, crises such as malnutrition, starvation, deforestation, and environmental destruction, conflict, and war will inevitably ensue.

The answer is development that gives rise to hope. Work; satisfactory compensation; adequate food, shelter, and health care; access to education—once these rights are ensured for all people, birth rates will fall into symmetry with death rates. The only way that such opportunity can be extended is sacrifice in standard of living and sharing by the overdeveloped, hyperaffluent world for the world in need. The suffering that the world would inflict can be offset only by absorbing, curing, caring, and suffering by individuals and nations that, because of the blessing of resourcefulness, can proffer help.

The provincial or local populational crisis of birth is related but somewhat different. Birth rates in western Europe, Canada, and the United States have slowed down to a ratio a bit above zero population growth. The problem is disproportionate expansion in some impoverished ethnic minority groups. In Germany nearly 50 percent of births are to alien workers, primarily from Turkey. In England, the same ratio is seen in nonwhite (black, Indian, and Asian) populations. In America we now have two scenarios: the white middle-class population for the most part enjoys stable birth rates, although in the Yuppie and DINK (double income, no kids) communities, raising families has pretty much fallen out of fashion. Meanwhile, among the black and Chicano communities, birth rates remain strong, especially for unmarried mothers. One can see why the cries of racism and genocide are heard when global and local population-control measures are proposed.

The answer, though, is exactly the same. It is not a triage or let-them-starve ethic. The let-nature-take-its-course ethic and the withdrawal-in-apathy ethic which are almost completely dominant today both evade responsibility and fail to enter into the suffering-redemption drama which is the moral meaning of human existence. Encouragement, assistance at some sacrifice to those of us who have so much, opportunity mainly in the economic and spiritual spheres—this is the surest policy for amelioration of the domestic population crisis. We need to learn the simple ecological lesson of feedback reaction. If we help those who hurt, even at a significant cost, we will be rewarded by peace and a sense of justice served and the delight of seeing prosperity come to our fellows. If we refuse to fund programs of assistance, education, maternal care, job training, and economic development, we will pay it out perhaps twofold in welfare costs, medicaid for the poor, and costs of police forces and prisons.

What is required is the renaissance of the virtue of mimesis, the ritual enactment of nature's own providence, justice, and nondiscrimination. An ecological ethic, enriched by all other components of our system, refined of its harshness by higher orders of moral conviction, can alone help us through this suffering. Mimesis, or ecological activity, can take the form of preservation or consumption. To chasten this natural value with a sense of urgency so that we must watch and wait requires that we move to the apocalyptic perspective and so on through the system until we reach the ultimate bearing of an eschatological ethic.

This chapter ends with a note of warning. The people of Kenya on the east coast of Africa experience both the desperation and the hope of population crisis of ecological ethics. In this country where children are the glory of life, symbols of wealth and security, the time of reckoning has come. The average family has eight children, with families of ten to twenty in the villages not uncommon. As population increases 4 percent per year, the population is doubling in an eighteen-year time span. Said a family-planning worker, "If something isn't done, we die!" The crisis is presenting itself in dramatic and urgent fashion: the pressure on food is felt as farmland and woodland decreases. People flock to the cities, where all services—food, housing, and health care—are stretched to the breaking point. But in this land, where polygamy is still practiced and where women are often seen not in tender love and needing protection from suffering but as a mark of prosperity, the children they bear are the best hope of the land. Today, the young people are learning family planning and contraceptive usage in the schools and villages. Despite frantic opposition the children sing songs like "The Coil Won't Destroy Your Brain." The traditional sign of resignation, *sanamabunba* (it's up to God—he will decide), is now being transformed into "we will decide."[21] Perhaps out of reverence for life and respect for nature the young will turn to the old and the old to the young and a blessed future will avert the curse. We conclude with the apocalyptic, yet prophetic words which bring the Old Testament to its close: "Behold, I will send you Elijah the prophet before the coming of the great and dreadful day of the Lord: And he shall turn the heart of the fathers to the children, and the heart of the children to their fathers, lest I come and smite the earth with a curse" (Mal. 4:5–6).

2 Apocalyptic Ethics of Human Sexuality:

PLAGUE

... lest I come and smite the earth with a curse.

Mal. 4:6

"Smite the earth with a curse!" "How ridiculous!" Nature does not bestow reward or bring revenge like that. We all know that what we call nature—the physical universe—is orderly, predictable, and absolutely indiscriminate. Surely it follows Newton's serene laws. And judgment—the commendation of good and condemnation of evil—this is a moral and not a natural process. Atoms and molecules, microbes and animals, these follow their built-in, ordained, and yet random processes. "Mother nature" is as ridiculous a notion as "wrathful God"—or is it?

The disease AIDS has entered the human world through a

22

rupture in the ecology membrane. It may be a manifestation of ecological infidelity. Like population, AIDS is now a raging epidemiological crisis. AIDS has become a natality crisis as phases 1 and 2 (where homosexuals and then prostitutes and drug abusers were afflicted) now yields to phase 3, where newborns are victims. Ecological and epidemiological crisis is disruption of our covenant work in the natural and human world. "The AIDS pandemic," writes Harvard biologist Stephen Jay Gould, "an issue that may rank with nuclear weaponry as the greatest danger of our era, provides a more striking proof that mind and technology are not omnipotent and that we have not cancelled our bond to nature."[1]

But we have neglected that bond. We have been insensitive to nature's warning in our procrastination to get serious about AIDS. We did not heed the alarm that sounded from Africa more than two decades ago. The point of "inoculation" was scarcely noted on the global health surveillance screens. Even today our state of concern is far less than it should be because, like the population crisis, AIDS appeared first among the poor, blacks, Haitians, gays, drug abusers, prostitutes, and the other despised and forgotten persons in our world. It is out there—beyond the pale—outside the camp. We can wall it out, and indeed we may. Although blacks constitute only 12 percent of the U.S. population, they represent 25 percent of all adult cases, 50 percent of the cases in women, and 53 percent of the child cases.[2] The rupture of AIDS into our apathetic world has come at the thin point of membrane breakage, down in the pockets of acute pain where dereliction is raging response to our "I don't give a damn about you" kind of world.

In 1983, a conference "Ethics of AIDS" was held at the University of Illinois and the West Side Medical Center, which is now one of the treatment centers of this dreaded disease. Only a handful of people showed up at the conference, and very few viewed the situation with any alarm. Now the magnitude of the problem is at long last coming into focus. Most of the countries of the world now have cases, including the countries thought to be impenetrable, like China and Russia. As of mid-1987 there were 50,000 reported cases worldwide. Dr. Jonathan Mann of the World Health Organization projects that between 500,000 and 3 million people will develop AIDS by 1992. In the United States, Dr. James Curran of the Communicable Disease Center reports that 36,000 people have had AIDS and over 21,000 have already died from it. He estimates that between 1 and 1.5 million are now infected with the virus, a great portion of whom will die from it.[3] In New York City already the major cause of death in women between twenty and forty years old is AIDS. But alarm can be translated into moral indignation or smug satisfaction. Gould goes on to caution us when we moralize about plagues.

> We must also grasp the perspective of ecology and evolutionary biology and recognize, once we reinsert ourselves properly into nature, that AIDS represents the ordinary workings of biology, not an irrational or diabolical plague with moral meaning . . . AIDS is a natural phenomenon, one of a recurring class of pandemic diseases. Yes, AIDS may run through the entire population, and may carry off a quarter or more of us. Yet it may make no *biological* difference to Homo Sapiens in the long run: there will still be plenty of us left and we can start again. Evolution cares as little for its agents—organisms struggling for reproductive success—as physics cares for individual atoms of hydrogen in the sun. But *we* care. These atoms are our neighbors, our lovers, our children and ourselves. AIDS is a natural phenomenon and, potentially, the greatest natural tragedy in human history.[4]

It is indeed in the realm of relationships, not in sheer nature itself, that the moral dimension begins to arise. There is a fatality and blind amorality as ecology tells us what to do. But in apocalyptic perspective human responsibility plays into what happens in nature. Dr. Roy Schwartz, vice president for education of the AMA, finds that AIDS is "a political disease, a social, religious and moral disease. That make it more complex to manage. It is also a civil rights disease, and that is both the fascination and damnation of the disease, and what makes it so difficult to know what to do."[5] But nature itself is not a placid reality; it agonizes, as we have argued, and evokes moral sympathies. But as Gould might agree, it is in the connectedness and reciprocity in nature's web, in the delights of coherence and purpose and in the pains of disjunction and damage, that nature becomes a part of the human moral world. Nature's trauma is the reality of nature that has been called apocalyptic. Just as time can be viewed in two ways—as duration (*chronos*) and meaning (*kairos*)—space can be viewed as extension (*physics*) and meaning (*apocalypsis*).

Understood in this way, the coming into our life of pathologic AIDS as a disease we can call a moral crisis. AIDS represents a breach in the customary nonvirulence of the microbial world. We have come to expect that the microorganisms of the life-world will occupy their own niche, exert their specific generational vitality and their natural populational dynamics, and not reach out destructively into the rest of nature. AIDS may indeed be an unnatural intrusion into the stratum of human life, perhaps overwhelming the compromised host organism in the same way that natural, benign flora in the body become destructive to persons whose resistance is defective or compromised. Patients with SCID, cancer, and transplant patients whose bone marrow has been irradiated are examples of such host compromise.

One of Dr. Lawrence Altman's reports on AIDS to the *New York Times* indeed raises this possibility. It may be that a genetic flaw in a group of proteins called the *Gc* group in certain persons makes them vulnerable to the transmutation of a benign organism into a killer.[6] There might also be a genetically derived AIDS-specific lymphocyte killer in some people. We will need to study carefully persons who have been exposed to HIV (Human Immunodeficiency Virus) and have become infected, yet do not get sick or succumb to the disease. Then we will come to know the relationship of the host organism to the pathogen. Dr. Susumu Tonegawa, winner of the 1987 Nobel Prize in medicine, has shown the importance of amplification and diversification in the field of human antibodies. This important scientific inquiry may yield ameliorative knowledge for the AIDS crisis. If there is an inheritance factor in AIDS, the nature of the evil shifts from the basis of willing action to recognition of a deeper cosmic flaw that marks a fallen world. The proliferation of AIDS among the poor and the despised of the world also positions the evil more as an aspect of messianic persecution than of moral perversion. An enigmatic mystery is unfolding before us. Our response ought to be concern and care, not condemnation.

The fact that AIDS has exerted its virulence at the point where humans are behaving in morally questionable ways—homosexuality (especially compulsive and promiscuous homosexuality), contaminated-needle drug abuse, prostitution, and other aberrant human encounters where bodily fluids are exchanged in uncommon ways—gives rise to the moral approbrium that surrounds AIDS. One Vatican spokesperson has called AIDS a "natural sanction" against homosexuality. That innocent children (hemophiliacs), the unborn and newborn offspring of infected mothers, and innocent spouses are infected confounds this view and creates a different moral appraisal. The assumption of innocence and victimization yields a more concerted effort to help. As we have seen in the case of population, it is the interpretation we make of suffering and whether we deem a person worthy or blameworthy of suffering that attenuates or intensifies our moral response.

If certain genetic subtypes are vulnerable to this disease and others are not, an entirely different moral response will occur. For now, our evaluative response associates the disease with the licentious breakdown of what our moral tradition has affirmed as "the good life" or "the way of life" (chaste, faithful, monogamous, and heterosexual). This breakdown has flourished from the 1960s forward in America. New patterns of sexual behavior have unleashed the plagues which we gather under the rubric STDs (sexually transmitted diseases), which include syphillis, gonorrhea, PID (Pelvic Inflamatory Disease), chlamydia, and now AIDS.

The release of the licentious "do your own thing" ethic was preceded by a loss of vitality in the traditional biblical sex-ethic as it degenerated into a pathological puritanism. The story and film *Dr. Strangelove, or How I Learned to Love the Bomb* parodied, in the figure of U.S. Air Force Commander Jack D. Ripper, the paranoic fear that communist forces, fluoridation of water, and all the new things that scare us seek to deplete and contaminate our "vital bodily fluids." Such films and books—indeed, all the reactions and counterreactions to the "free-love" movement of the 1960s and 1970s—betray our concern that human sexual activity has gotten out of hand and must be shaped again by ethical commitments.

The AIDS crisis as a moral phenomenon invites us to consider the long-forgotten apocalyptic feature of reality and its point of entry into the moral soul. Apocalyptic is the word we give to a certain reality—or better, potentiality—of nature. Apocalyptic is to nature what we shall later see eschatology is to history in terms of moral force. It is also a mode of speech. There is an element of crisis and abrupt breakthrough or breakout in nature itself and to some extent in time and history. This physical and temporal disruption we call apocalyptic. There is also a special mode of language and literature which bears the same title. In one sense all of the various dimensions of ethics that we are identifying as parts of a comprehensive whole are, in fact, different manners of speech, ways that we give expression to the singular moral reality we experience.

THE APOCALYPTIC GENRE

In 1930 Shailer Mathews, theologian and dean of the University of Chicago's Divinity School, wrote a classic essay on apocalyptic literature in which he argued that the genre emerged to meet the specific expressive needs of a certain people in a given period of time.[7] He felt that apocalyptic literature united Babylonian myths and symbolism with the religious faith of the Jews, chastened by the Babylonian exile and expressed within Hellenistic culture. The genre thus has to do with impending judgment and deliverance. The symbolism, like the zodiac or other Babylonian myths, used natural elements (sun, moon, stars) and animals. This genre, like its precursor prophetism, encouraged faith, hope, and responsible waiting for deliverance by setting forth pictures of a future, revelations (apocalypsis) or visions of sheep, bulls, birds, belials, antichrists, all of which symbolized impending events, liberating and catastrophic. From the earliest texts in Persian and Zoroastrian religion down to our present flood of apocalyptic texts such as *The Late Great Planet Earth*, the following themes are found: belief in two cosmic powers (good and evil) and belief in two distinct ages—the present, which is under the sway of the evil one, and the eternal age of God's kingdom, which is breaking in to conquer this present evil age. The general moods of expectancy and dread, polar dispositions in the face of the unknown and mystery, have fashioned and in turn are fashioned by apocalyptic.

Some of the apocalyptic classics of ancient Judaism, Greece, and primitive Christianity (the genre flourished from the fourth century B.C. to the first century A.D.) are the Old Testament books Joel and Daniel, Er's vision of the next world in Plato's *Republic*, Mark 13, and the Book of Revelation. A famous text shaped by apocalyptic vision is Paul's 1 Corinthians 15.

> If in this life only we have hope in Christ, we are of all men most miserable. But now is Christ risen from the dead, and become the firstfruits of them that slept. For since by man came death, by man came also the resurrection of the dead. For as in Adam all die, even so in Christ shall all be made alive. But every man in his own order: Christ the firstfruits; afterward they that are Christ's at his coming. Then cometh the end, when he shall have delivered up the kingdom to God, even the Father; when he shall have put down all rule and all authority and power. For he must reign, till he hath put all enemies under his feet. The last enemy that shall be destroyed is death. For he hath put all things under his feet. But when he saith all things are put under him, it is manifest that he is excepted, which did put all things under him. And when all things shall be subdued unto him, then shall the Son also himself be subject unto him that put all things under him, that God may be all in all. (Vv. 19–28)

Among the elements we note in this passage are, first, the conflict between the great forces of good and evil which in this resurrection context are the forces of life, death, and eternal life. Second
is the note that the realities of that unseen, envisioned, eternal
world are continuous with this world. "If in this life *only* we have
hope. . . ." Apocalypses are not fantastic projections, desperate longings of deprived persons for a world they wish could be. Rather, they
are extrapolations of what could be from what is. Apocalypse can
also be seen as receptions from the world as it will be back into the
world that is. Apocalypse is a deeper look into nature with blinders
and cataracts removed.

Third is the moral aspect. As in all apocalyptic texts, time and
beyond-time, nature and supernature, are involved with the end
purpose of moral instruction. This present age—evil and wasting
away—has a corrupting and contaminating lure on those human beings who are living through it. It is not accidental that, in the history of art and literature, images of corruption of the flesh have
often been associated with the plagues: leprosy, bubonic plague, tu-
berculosis, cancer, and now AIDS. But the divine King whose kingdom
has broken into this world has already started to defeat the powers
of sickness, death, and evil. In rabbinic pictures the coming Messiah
is seen sitting among the lepers at the gate of the city. In Isaiah 35
the impending (apocalyptic) highway of God is one where nature
erupts in healing—the lame walk, and the blind see. In Isaiah 53
the redeeming Messiah is cast in the visage of an afflicted leper:
"Despised and rejected . . . we could not bear to look upon him . . .
he bore our diseases" (vv. 3–4). This new kingdom belongs to the
righteous, those who have put aside the dark world with its lures
and have joined the King to go into that realm of loss and corruption in order to absorb, suffer, rescue, heal, and redeem.

APOCALYPSE IN NATURE

But now a tough question confronts us. Does this symbolic language of apocalyptic in any way depict reality? Does apocalyptic expression tell us about the way the world really is? In this literature
and the oral tradition behind it, we have normative, not descriptive,
language about reality. Stephen Jay Gould misses the point by requiring that normative language be descriptive; otherwise, for him,
it is fanciful and dangerous. To his point, it must be said that reality
is rich and multifaceted. Real objects and events cannot be de-

scribed in just one language, such as the language of empirical ob-
servation. Reality must be described in a wide variety of descriptive,
prescriptive, and normative languages, all of which have the power
to convey particular facets of truth. In one sense AIDS is an event
in nature amenable to scientific discernment and ultimately explained, in Gould's words, by "a mechanism." In another sense, the
phenomenon is explained by apocalyptic speech which is in part descriptive, at least in its catastrophic aspect, but is ultimately more
dualistic, explaining what is going on in terms of what has gone
wrong and why it is happening. Apocalyptic is a purposive throb at
the heart of nature. It is rupture and crisis which are leading somewhere. Gould says there is no place for this language of meaning. If
we follow his descriptive thesis to its logical conclusion, there is
nothing wrong or grievous about AIDS—it just is.

In contrast to this positivist and empiricist view of nature, we
find that the Judeo-Christian view of nature and history attempts
through apocalyptic eyes to see meaning in epidemics and pandem-
ics. Speaking of the Jews who bequeathed this tradition to civilization, Paul Johnson writes that "no people has ever insisted more
firmly that history has a purpose and humanity a destiny." That
there was a providential purpose and a divine scheme for the human race and that this involved dimensions of personal being, sexuality, human relations, and family life was a belief that Judaism
"clung to with heroic persistence in the face of savage suffering."[8]

The constitutive event for the people who became Israel was
rescue from plague and exodus from bondage. The memory of natural cataclysm from the delivery amid plagues to the opening of the
waters at the Sea of Reeds firmly established in the moral soul
shaped by this heritage an expectancy or conversely a dread at what
nature offered if the people lived in affirmation or abandonment of
"the way" or "the light." This way of life, this Torah which is the
light of life, was associated with Moses and Sinai. "Moses," writes
Johnson, "was a Jewish Archetype. . . . He was a prophet and a
leader . . . a man of intense spirituality, loving solitary communion
with himself and God in the remote countryside, seeing visions and
epiphanies and apocalypses."[9]

In this puritan and prophylactic spirit of Hebrew prophetism,
Cotton Mather, the first significant figure in American medicine,
saw diphtheria and smallpox as outbreaks of divine judgment recalling the people to faithfulness and uprightness. Apocalyptic perception enables one to see in nature what is concealed from normal
vision. A cloud pillar is just a cumulus formation, a plague of lo-

custs just a nuisance to eyes from which the apocalyptic blindfold has not been raised. The major intellectual crisis of the twentieth century, a crisis which precipitates the moral crisis, is that which denies that the unseen world is "real." Empiricism and positivism say that the real is that which can be seen, touched, and measured. The radical break that Western culture has made with both the Hebraic-Christian and Platonic traditions of the unseen and ideal reality has made us skeptical about meaning and purpose, therein gravely compromising our spiritual and moral capacity.

Apocalyptic is a part of complete ethical conscience for both natural and supernatural reasons. In terms of nature alone we experience the aspect of disruption and discontinuity in space and time. This amplitude we call apocalyptic. Theologically we have accepted apocalyptic as part of our picture of moral reality since Jesus accepted the baptism of John on the Jordan. This submission to that understanding of "kingdom come" gives apocalyptic an enduring validity.

What do we know about dread and expectancy, the receptor sites of apocalypses in the human soul? In what sense are these capacities part of normal spiritual and moral intelligence? The *Oxford English Dictionary* traces the word *dread* back through its etymological journey in English speech and finds that it combines the meanings of fear and reverence. It is "awful" fear.[10] It is also the seat of "awful" or "wonderful" expectancy. The expectancy of natural miracle, salutary transformation of natural processes, and deliverance is one side of apocalyptic conscience. Conversely, the dread of natural calamity, not blind indiscriminate tragedy like an earthquake or predictable tragedy like aging and dying, but specific, surprising, yet sensible calamity activates this faculty of the moral soul.

Moral attitudes and actions in turn proceed from this component of the psyche. The attitude or posture of waiting, watching, being there, and remaining is one response. Dr. Rieux in Camus's *The Plague* and Father Damien among the lepers of Molokai are living features who embody this posture. "Nonetheless, he [Dr. Rieux] knew that the tale he had to tell . . . could be only the record of . . . what assuredly would have to be done again in the never-ending fight against terror and its relentless onslaughts, despite their personal afflictions, by all who, while unable to be saints but refusing to bow down to pestilences, strive their utmost to be healers."[11] Saints and healers abide amid threat. The quality they embody is a subtle but powerful willingness to take a risk, to participate in trial, and to bear pain and suffering with another.

The contrary posture, the negentropic as opposed to the tropic apocalyptic ethic, is repulsion, disregard, and withdrawal. In *The Normal Heart*, a drama on AIDS, the police, the ambulance driver, and even the mortician refuse to come near, to touch, or to identify with the victim. But this is the expected response to the "awful." Rudolf Otto (*The Idea of the Holy*) showed how an awesome experience, the primal perception of mystery, evokes both attraction and repulsion, both endearment and dread.

AIDS AS APOCALYPSE

The AIDS crisis is provoking this kind of ambivalent challenge today within our moral souls. The call to help and draw near is the call to alleviate if possible—but if not, to abide in the presence of suffering. This means first doing everything we can to prevent the occurrence of AIDS. This means nurturing wholesome life-styles, ways of life in accord with the prophylactic ethics of our tradition. It means fostering vigorous educational programs and emergency prophylaxis in a world we know has gone astray. It means drawing near in support when the disease strikes. This last measure of sharing suffering entails funding research, supporting nondiscriminative and nonretaliative policies in the workplace, at school, and in public services. It also prompts us to find ways to provide AZT and other costly medications for all who need them, making available excellent clinical care and finally ensuring dignified terminal and hospice care. In sum, an ethical response which resonates with the noble side of an apocalyptic ethic will attack the crisis, not turn its back in disgust and withdraw.

Three moral characteristics of an apocalyptically tempered ethic that will serve us throughout the coming decades of the AIDS crisis will be (1) thoughtful patience at the inception of this dread pandemic, (2) grave seriousness about the potency of sex in this world that has made it so casual, and (3) the careful yet serene preparation for the Armageddon-like struggle that faces us.

Often an apocalypse can be averted or blunted in its force. The AIDS epidemic may be demolished in its tracks by a powerful prophylactic vaccination or sophisticated therapy. New research breakthroughs in the coming years may make this possible. This dramatic rescue, however, is unlikely. We will probably need the grace of waiting, thoughtful patience at the outset of this pandemic to demolish its devastation as much as is possible.

In an important article exploring the modifications to behavior that are occurring among the homosexual community in response to the AIDS alarm, Peter Davis writes: "Since it is primarily contracted through sex and the use of drugs, two activities associated both with desire and freewill, AIDS tests us as no disease ever has. It is the first plague in the history of mankind whose regulation is entirely dependent upon our knowing behavior."[12] As one commentator said, "Thousands of lives have been lost *needlessly.*"

Three relatively untested powers of the moral psyche are challenged by the AIDS crisis. Some people know they do not have the disease. They may feel smug, even gleeful, at the misfortune of others or at best cautious about themselves, their relationship with others, and the provision of a safer society for their fellows. There are many people, however, who do not know whether or not they have been infected or whether they will succumb to the disease. These exhibit a new disease called "Afraids." This unusual state of apprehension—not knowing for sure whether one has been exposed and has not yet developed antibodies, not knowing whether the infection will show up on later screening, or, if one has been tested positive, not knowing what is going to happen—this veiled ignorance is an unprecedented experience in human psychology. There is a third group that has the disease and knows that death is inevitable, though perhaps it can be delayed. Here the virtues of accommodation and acceptance are called for. This strength of endurance requires the added grace of accepting guilt and bearing the additional shame that others heap on us in their rage and fear.

Gould has rightly noted that this pandemic both shows us how much of life is within our rational and technical control and how much remains beyond our control. By its very nature apocalyptic ethics is decisional challenge in the face of the unknown. Here we face mystery in the uncertainty as to what will happen and obscurity about what it means, all undergirded by the fear of judgment and hope for deliverance. Apocalypse calls for empathetic ethics.

Often in the face of such an unpredictable future, those who are afflicted *panic,* run to some refuge thought to be safe, or even commit suicide. The more becoming posture, true to our own nature and faithful to reality as we know it, is that of *patience.* The moral imperative activating patience involves active watching and searching for ways out—ways to ameliorate existent suffering and avoid that which is coming.

As a second aspect of an apocalyptic ethic, the AIDS crisis is causing us to become acutely aware, as were our primitive fore-bears, of the awesome potency of sexual power. Davis continues:

> In the kingdom of AIDS [an apocalyptic image], a penis itself, often linked to a sword in folktales [a smoking gun in current political parlance], again becomes a deadly weapon. . . . Since our perception of threat presumably determines our behavior, perhaps only an exaggerated depiction of the danger AIDS now poses for heterosexuals will prevent that worse-case scenario from ultimately becoming the reality. It seems paradoxical; but the result is we are being warned that we are all bombs and some of our fuses have been lighted.[13]

In a world where images of potency have been emasculated and dis-placed by casual and technical images, this renewed perception comes as a shock. Actually the whole field of perinatal science— genetics, fertilization, cloning, and related areas—opens up in a new way the tremendous potency of life, including germinal cells and sexuality. It recalls us to a long-lost dimension of our moral self.

In the primitive and ancient world the awesome potency of sex-ual power became the basis for comparing one's potency and fertil-ity with the very creative power of the gods. The moral significance of the analogy or participation was to exert the power with awe-some respect. The strictures against misguided and perverted sex (turned away from proper goals) emerged from this sublime sense that human recreation and procreation was in some sense identified with the divine potency. We now know both the deliterious mi-crobes that voyage along the conjugal channels (AIDS) and the "good viruses" that may indeed safeguard against disease. Both open new vistas of sexual responsibility. In Karl Barth's ethics we see the profound consequence of this awesome wonder about our sexual be-ing which draws to itself both ecstasy and shame. Barth identifies the *imago Dei*, the most central spiritual and moral capacity of the soul, with male and female love: "In the image of God created he him, male and female created he them" (Gen. 1:27).

Third, an apocalyptic mood of ethics fosters a readiness to en-dure a long struggle of good and evil, hope and disappointment. The symbols of an agonizing, intractable conflict in which a people are sustained by the expectation of deliverance are apocalyptic symbols, perfectly pertinent to the AIDS ordeal (see Isaiah 40).

Immediate moral quandaries about AIDS press for attention. Shall testing be required or only offered? Shall records be kept confidential? Shall public interests override personal liberties? Shall infected or diseased persons lose their rights to certain protections? Shall experimental drugs be made available faster by circumventing research regulations? Shall resuscitation be offered or withheld from AIDS patients who arrest? All these and myriad other issues are subsumed and directed by the more basic issues of a society's fundamental commitment.

The medical profession in its internal ethics has struggled with the ethics of sustaining care in the face of danger. In 1847, when the first AMA code was published, a small companion booklet held that, during epidemics, it was the physician's duty "to face the danger, and to continue their labors for the alleviation of the suffering, even at the jeopardy of their own lives."[14]

This document, growing out of the pastoral commitments of medicine in the early nineteenth century (e.g. Percival's Code), was clinically naive in its knowledge about antisepsis and asepsis, since there were not adequate antimicrobial agents and prophylactics at that time. But to its credit the document reflects a compassion for the sick and a willingness to suffer and die for another (even by holding near someone who is contaminated) that emerges out of the more palpable religious faith of the period. When we witness Catholic sisters caring for the sick at complete disregard for their own protection or read of Father Damien beginning his sermon one morning on Molokai with the words "my fellow lepers," we are reminded of an ethic now alien from our self-protecting and pragmatic world.

For some time the AMA code was silent on the ethics of exposure and risk. At the end of 1986, the AMA issued a statement on physicians' responsibilities toward patients with AIDS which reflects the more libertarian ethos of our time. While the document acknowledged the long history of self-sacrifice in the presence of suffering and the historic commitment to be with contagious patients, it counseled, "A physician shall, in the provision of appropriate patient care, except in emergencies, be free to choose whom to serve."[15] This swing of position reflects a basic change in the moral mandate of medicine which is shaped by internal professional conscience and external societal requirement. Following serious critique of this position, the Council of Ethical and Judicial Affairs of the AMA has reaffirmed the traditional "stay in there" position. As the profession continues to struggle with the conflicts of its entrepreneurial and civil-service character with the more historic charter of sacrificial ministry, the AIDS crisis will clarify the fundamental commitments of medicine and nursing.

In 1987 President Reagan pledged before the National Institutes of Health that he would do all that is in "God's power to defeat this disease" that had struck down the little black children in the hospital ward he recently visited. "We will continue to fight until we have put it away as we did polio and smallpox." This commendable spirit of commitment is exactly what is needed, since we are dealing not only with a virus and a vulnerable host but also with principalities and powers of evil: hatred, homophobia, retribution, guilt, shame, and sin. We are dealing with structures and systems of evil as well as collectivities and serendipities of good.

Finally, one reservation about the apocalyptic mode of ethical analysis must be mentioned. Though apocalyptic speech demands secrecy, we must not succumb to that demand. The author of an apocalypse is always a pseudonym—an Ezekiel, an Enoch, or just the seer. One does not pronounce the name of the Holy One. We use the unutterable tetragrammaton YHWH. Those who flirt with the devil can never remember his name. But now our visions, warfare, and ultimate victory must be open and accessible. For the sake of those who will be wounded and those who will suffer, die, and be disfigured and transfigured, our efforts must be revealed. Nemesis and deliverance hover over us. Ethics therefore must be apocalyptic, broken open and revealed. In our civilization's conscience the ultimate apocalyptic image is the image of a kingdom and a banquet table. Here persons come from east and west, north and south—the great and the small, the distinguished and the despised—all who have passed through great tribulation. The table is exclusive, yet all tribes and all peoples are welcome, for all are the subjects of the intense, searching love of that King, that host (Revelation 7).

3 Biologic Ethics of Attraction and Affection:

BEING SEXUAL

The family requires the most delicate mixture of nature and convention, of human and divine, to subsist and perform its function. Its base is merely bodily reproduction, but its purpose is the formation of civilized human beings.

Allan Bloom, *The Closing of The American Mind*

The breakdown of the family will make experimental breeding possible.

B. F. Skinner, *Walden II*

Nature, Mr. Olnar, is what we are put in this world to rise above.

Kathryn Hepburn to Humphrey Bogart, in *The African Queen*

The community we sense in apocalyptic vision we also know in our genes. We did not need AIDS to show us that we are confused and confounded about our sexual being and our relationships. The family is now caught in a profound crisis. Whereas ecological ethics ask of us engaged participation and apocalyptic ethics urgent contact, the biologic ethics of human bonding invite enduring commitment through time and tribulation. The adaptive genius of the family across biologic history is found in the support and succor it offers in a threatening world. In terms of the attachment/detachment dialectic created by our response to suffering, family life

36

brings out in us the capacity to endure vexation for the sake of transmitting to others a world intact and perhaps enriched. Family and community are bastions against the terrors of life. At their best they are havens of peace from the perpetual turmoil all around, safe places for propagation and edification.

Crises in nature and history put the family to the test. When the body is badly injured, for example, spouses split and families disintegrate in predictable relation to the severity of the disgrace. Very few families survive quadriplegia. As far as time and history are concerned, many studies have pointed out the impact of war on family structure. Some go as far as to argue that sexual and familial values were irrevocably altered by World War II.[1] The arrival of antibiotics and an apocalyptic atmosphere combined to create an ethos where fear of infection, detection, and conception no longer kept one chaste. Spatial (aesthetic) or temporal (chronic) disruptions inevitably affect our patterns of living together.

This chapter is concerned with the practical issue of sexual being, being male and female and being together in love and familial bond. We live in this way not only by natural inclination but also for the sake of saying that life shall go on. After this chapter deals with being together, the next intimately related chapter will consider the theme of being with child.

CRISIS IN BEING AND BEING TOGETHER

We have argued that humans are called to be together in the midst of life's crises and that this being together (being with another) is the very nature of our personal being. In our discussion of apocalypse we noted that covenant is a human response to surrounding peril. The Noachic covenant, for example, is a bonding relationship with God, nature (e.g. the animal world), and family. In Paul Ramsey's discussion "Genetic Apocalypse and the End of Man,"[2] he argues against the genetic apocalypticists who contend that we are so polluting our genetic being that one day "there will be none like us to come after us." Ramsey retorts that the biblical covenant of life-with-life both ridicules the question (why arrogantly assume that those who follow should be just like us?) and commands that our being and our life together be committed not to annihilate the future but to offer it the sacrifice of our flesh. In biologic ethics stewardship of the body is basic to human responsibility. Happy fulfillment of the inner purposes of our being and faithfulness to the God who gives life to us is our fundamental destiny, second only to the primary vocation of knowing and glorifying God even if this life should fail.

The crisis in which we find ourselves leads many to see only sheer absurdity in the foregoing affirmation. Christopher Lasch, who has carefully studied the modern experience of narcissism and of family tribulation, argues that the capacity to look beyond—to memory, community, or possibility—is nearly obliterated in the human soul.

The crisis is one where we have lost our sense about who we are and who we were given to the world to be. The collapse of a clear and compelling sense of nature and destiny has left us floundering, taking enormous toll in all aspects of our life but particularly devastating our sense of biosexual, parental, and familial self.

The film *The Witches of Eastwick* attempts to expose this void we feel in the relational self by conjuring up with the techniques of witches' brew and the old magic manual *Malleus Maleficarum* the spiritual forces of evil and good. In the story three young women, all divorced and somewhat concerned about the loneliness and dullness that stalk their lives, conjure up old diabolo himself, typecast Jack Nicholson, portraying Darrell Van Horn. In a beautiful scene graced by a John Williams sound track, he asks each women what is going on in her "heart of hearts." They respond with recital of the great human woes that always invite the wiles of the devil: "It's a short life—it starts when you open your eyes and you see everything moving faster and faster"; "Me—I always see snakes—they crawl all over—hundreds and hundreds of them"; and "It's the pain that scares me."

The passage seems to draw from the famous text of Freud in *Civilization and Its Discontents:* "Suffering comes from three quarters: from our own body, which is destined to decay and dissolution and cannot even dispense with anxiety and pain as danger-signals; from the outer world, which can rage against us with the most powerful and pitiless forces of destruction; and finally from our relationships with other men. The unhappiness which has this last origin we find perhaps more painful than any other."[3] The frustrations of transiency, palpable evil, and pain provoke in our inner being and relational self one of these responses: to collapse into apathy and monotony, to seek the lures of temptation which promise vibrancy of life at such a small price (one's soul), or to venture the life of trusting responsibility and the communion of suffering and care.

The crisis that surrounds us today is complicated by the fascinating lures and distractions of an affluent "create it and sell it" kind of world. The classic and biblical heritage, the song and story of life's meaning, has been muted to a faint whisper. Myriad other forces join to obscure the vision of who we are and what in God's name (or the devil's) we are here for.

The failed vision is most grievous as we seek to express our sexual and relational self. The technologies of bioscience also come into play: surely the contraceptive and sterilization technologies have offered us the freedom of reconceiving ourselves as sexual beings. The array of new modes of baby making—though still of miniscule importance on a national, to say nothing of the global, scale—do have some impact on our self-concept and the perception of ourselves as conjugal and procreative beings. Of 3.7 million babies born in 1986, only 100 involved surrogate mothers; 500 were conceived in petri dishes; and somewhere between 8,000 and 20,000 came into being through artificial insemination. In addition to this there were 1,650,000 abortions during that year.[4] Yet the influence of these innovations on our values and ways of blending lives is not great.

A far more tangible and powerful influence on our sense of ourselves as persons is the widespread experience of divorce. Many of this generation have lived through the divorce of their own parents and expect the same pain and expense for themselves if they decide to become married. Anyone who offers marriage, divorce, or family therapy today knows how widespread this occurrence and fear is. Other influences assert themselves such as the Western welfare-state nations making provisions for retirement of their citizens, so that persons need not produce children to ensure old-age security. Other sociological challenges—urbanization, mobility, separation of families across the country, and working demands—may also have an influence. First we must explore the biologic influences on our singleness and togetherness.

THE BIOLOGY OF ETHICS

When two human beings came together today and find it desirable yet extremely difficult to be together, they are experiencing energies of affection and attraction, aggression and repulsion, which proceed from our very basic genetic and biologic nature. Though the capacity for friendship and intimacy is, of course, shaped through social influences and enabled by acts of emotion, thought, and will, the original impulses to affection, attachment, bonding, and love are born in our biologic substance. Recent scholarship in biologic ethics has shown the great beauty and power of this moral part of us. Let us review in three stages these findings and their bearing on the character of our sexual-relational being. First, we take note of *evolutionary ethics*. Second, note the moral insights that emerge in the science of human *ethology*. Finally, we mention what might be called *extrapolate ethical theory* in its general thrust as well as its concrete bearing on our being as sexual and mating creatures.

Naturalistic and *evolutionary ethics* is a very ancient line of thought, emerging with the first philosopher who saw the flux or movement within the processes of nature and in the passage of life between generations. The notion that life rises and falls like a mist in evening and morning, like the blazing and vibrant yet fragile wildflowers, becomes a normative sense about how things are meant to be. It remains the task of the evolutionists of the nineteenth century, thinkers like Charles Darwin, to note the flowing, developing patterns of adaptation, selection, mutation, and change and to begin a discussion of the goods and evils inherent in the processes of the evolution of life forms.

One of the first values/disvalues noted relates to the impetus to survive. It appears that all organisms, including humans, have a built-in need to send life on to another generation and so to ensure the survival of their genes. A certain nobility surrounds this instinct. At one level there is the desire for survival, the yearning to perpetuate oneself. Taken to the extreme, this impulse would not seem to encourage the bearing of offspring who would sap life from parents and succeed them when they have passed on. Yet in biologic wisdom, purely self-oriented impulses of immortality yield to the finer values of giving life to others, perhaps even at the cost of one's own life.

One of the loveliest metaphors for this generous animus in the brute kingdom is also expressed in one of the most profound of theological themes. When religion recites the cathartic hymn of forgiveness "washed in the blood of the lamb," it is recalling one such ritual. In a flock of sheep it sometimes happens that the newborn lamb of one mother dies at birth while the mother of another dies giving birth. Now the flock faces the double tragedy of a childless mother who will pine and an orphan lamb who will die. Since they are not blood related, they will not naturally join their tragic fates redemptively. However, if the orphan lamb is washed in the blood of the mother, it will call forth an attraction, and the bereft mother will take the orphan as her own. This evolutionary precursor of human adoption is rooted in the even more fundamental impulse impulse of safeguarding continuity, albeit under the guise of blood immortality.

Related to such nurture, another evolving biologic ethic is altruism. Jane Goodall observed cases at the Gombe Stream National Park in Tanzania where older siblings assumed care for orphaned chimpanzee infants. This rudimentary form of the gesture, which bears no self-benefit and perhaps even entails hardship, is heightened in human self-sacrifice for friends or colleagues (family or fellow soldiers in war). The ultimate act of agapic love, Jesus of Nazareth's laying down of his life, brings into relief several other elements inherent in the altruistic act, including the appropriation into oneself of others' suffering and the bearing in one's own sacrificial body of the evil that necessitates generic suffering and the potential of redemption. While Edward O. Wilson, a Harvard zoologist, says that the expected apotheosis or the artifice of eternity sullies the act of martyrdom, we would respond that it holds as a virtuous act, since in the face of God the suicide or homicide may not be deemed noble.

The social Darwinists looked closely at the evolution of species into Homo Sapiens; observed predatory, survivalist, and exploitive behavior; and posited a capitalistic ethos, emergent in nature where the strong live and thrive at the expense of the weak. The "eat or be eaten" ethic enhances the pleasure of some by inflicting pain on others. Here we have a value that shows all of the ambiguity of most biologically driven values.

We might expect refinement of virtue across the span of evolution. Power could build up into genuine service. We find, on the other hand, that aggression and enterprise as qualities have the two-edged capacity to help or harm. Aggression takes us into the realm of ethologic values.

Biologic values may be identified as *ethological* as well as evolutionary. Here we look more at the structure of existence than at behaviors that evolve through time. Great animal ethologists like Konrad Lorenz have looked at the instincts and very primal modes of behavior in various species, including humans, and related these to our reflections about good and evil, right and wrong. Lorenz entitled one of his early works *Das Sogennante Böse* (The so-called evil); Wickler followed with a volume entitled *The Biology of the Ten Commandments*.[5] Numerous authors have shown the biologic basis for virtues and vices, sins and good deeds, some arguing reductively that genes and instincts determine all behavior, others seeing a continuum of impulse up through the levels of one's being.

Aggression, as it becomes the basis of libido as a psychic force, is the primary ethological quality possessing moral importance. The drive toward satisfaction, toward a sustained hedonic level, even toward the higher achievements of creativity and generosity, are, of course, fundamental to ethics. Though narcissism is related to aggression and hedonic drive, it is also a gentler, somewhat countervailing impulse. It leads one to the excesses of self-absorption and neglect of interhumanity; it also serves the salutary purposes of drawing inward in self-grooming and protective care of oneself and one's own. The fact that most ethics extol self-respect and self-love as a precondition of care for others shows the virtue of this impulse.

Another ethological value pertinent to our particular concern of sexual and procreative being is that of the family bond. Peter Singer argues that natural tendencies such as "kin selection" and family bond can and do become the basis for rules of human behavior. "Fostering family bonds means that children, the sick, and the aged get better care than they would from an imperial bureaucracy, or if they had to rely on the broad altruistic impulses of strangers."[6] When these innate tendencies are cleansed from certain unfortunate ethnocentric elements, they can become rules and guides that serve the good of the whole.

Sometimes we need to be called beyond the level of the animal we are and rise to higher levels of controlled appetite, deferred gratification, and altruism. At other times we need to be drawn back into our animal nature in its simple celebration, its authenticity and playfulness. Plato argued that we could resort to animal impulses and yet not succumb to barbarism. The passions, driven by the genetic, biologic, and endocrinal substructure of our being, can sublimate and serve the nobler purposes of enhancing and enriching life, or they can drive downward in destructive or autistic fury.

Biologic impulse is premoral. It has the potential to be transformed into virtue, now defined not as brute strength but as human excellence or even divine grace. In this sense an ethical system that works as a continuum of value such as we have proposed is further justified. The authentic realization of any dimension of value and the proper functioning of any function of the soul requires that the given level be chastened by cognate levels of ethics. Normative biologism, for example, in order to be free from the ethical heresy of vitalism, must be founded and activated by apocalyptic and ecological virtue. It must also be driven toward psychic, social, rational, and ultimately eschatological meanings. Each virtue, to be true to itself, must be deepened by its precursors and elevated by its successors.

A final spectrum of biologic values that bears on our natality exploration might be called *extrapolated* values, or what Don Campbell calls scientific-mediational values.[7] These values are social constructs or artifacts that can be affirmed by moral reason because they make sense out of what we have learned from the biosphere's wisdom. If we are true to the biologic foundations of our being, we ought to provide rational justification for the innate behavior of eliminating war, resisting genocide, reducing poverty and overpopulation, maintaining the ozone shield, and requiring clean and wholesome air, water, food, and habitat. These obvious and necessary extrapolates of being in the life-world are essential requirements of the biologic ethic.

The composite wisdom of biologic ethics in its evolutionary, ethological, and extrapolated insights is seldom presented in such an articulate manner as it has been in the work of Edward O. Wilson. In his award-winning book *On Human Nature*, he draws on the biologic and anthropological sciences to reflect on the power, meaning, and raison d'être of sex in human beings. Sex, he claims, is not designed primarily for reproduction. Evolution has much more efficient ways of cloning, budding, and replicating if that were the central purpose. Nor is the primary goal that of achieving and affording pleasure. "The vast majority of animal species perform the sexual act mechanically and ... sex is in every sense a gratuitously consuming and risky activity." Why, then, has sex evolved? Why have we become sexual and mating beings? "The principal answer is that sex creates diversity. And diversity is the way a parent hedges its bets against an unpredictably changing environment."[8]

We are called back to our original thesis. We are attracted to one another and commit ourselves to another in moral response to surrounding and impending crises. Life's drama of suffering, death, and transfiguration becomes more bearable when shared—indeed, the moral commitment between two people mediates suffering and channels help. In our moral being we strive to be less apathetic and more empathetic and sympathetic. This is what it means to be morally alive. In our actions we seek to alleviate hurt and the causes of hurt and to offer help. Loving one another tones down the agony of uncertainty and the trauma of tragedy. It also prepares us to make enduring rather than transient commitments. By mediating the eternal (God is love), pain-sharing love redeems the treachery of space and time, the inescapable conditions of our existence.

Human sexual bonding as an anthropological phenomenon also engenders this union amid crises and threats of alienation and annihilation. As such it serves as the ultimate expression of biologic ethics in the service of our sexual being and being together. Though disrupting and disorienting forces continually challenge the stability of partnership, other fundamental forces hold it together. Among these forces are the development in evolution of the menstrual as opposed to the estral cycle. This serves to extend sexual excitability across the entire course of life and receptivity over almost the entirety of the sexual period. Pugh mentions two other enticements toward enduring companionship: the development of a female orgasm, and an intensification of the emotional element in the human sexual embrace. The intense emotional content of the human embrace may be the result of retaining the infantile emotional response to clinging.[9]

Stability is introduced by nature into human sexual life, both for the enhancement of life and for propagation. Only in adequate peace and security can we pass life on. We embrace and hold on to each other throughout this precipitous night. By this hold we affirm that life shall prevail over death and that good shall ultimately triumph.

But basic and formidable as the biologic directive is, shaping our being, relationships, and behaviors with silent but awesome force, it cannot stand alone. Its insufficiency is made whole only as joined to the companion virtues which we explore throughout this book.

ETHICAL ASPECTS OF SEXUAL BEING

The relevance of the biologic vector of ethics enhanced in power by the accompanying continuum of value becomes vivid when we discuss a few representative perinatal moral issues that bear on sexual being and mating behavior. A first series of issues has to do with gender, male and female. The truth about male and female, man and woman, holds together the mystery of these two values—attraction and affection. The doctrine of difference and complementarity checks the dangers of homogeneity in the equality doctrine. An affinity doctrine, stressing equality and liberty, checks the exploitative potential of a differentiation doctrine.

Although we have some reason to believe that matriarchy and feminine ascendency was present in early human evolution (primitive religions focus on earth mothers, for example), earliest traditions seem to be marked by male dominance and authority which created the patterns of provision and protection over the wife and children. This dominion was not crass and exploitative; rather, it grew out of the natural inclination of genuine affection and fidelity. For modern people this has become a problem.

In recent years, the needs of freedom and equality have led all persons of good will to cleanse the extant practice of male dominance of its harmful qualities and restore a rightful reciprocity between the sexes. The salutary impulse of a father shielding mother and children from harm had to be separated from a paternalism that protected others from taking the risks that creative living and maturation required. Subordination, based on strength rather than right, also had to go. Yet it remained true that, in an ethos where shared suffering yielded liberation, it did make sense for the male to take upon himself the burden of providing for his family amid a cutthroat world while the woman bore, as was her unique gift, the burden of child nurture and of maintaining the domestic economy. "The woman," said a 1920s Chicago gangster in an unusual flash of insight, "is the educator of husband and family." The good families I have observed are communities which nurture but do not stifle their members in overprotection. When a child is able, he or she starts to share burdens and responsibilities. The perspective of care is always driven from the starting point of caring for one's own—out to neighbors and community and then out to the large global society. Such families are places where pain can be borne redemptively. To thrive, the young need sacrificial patience and attention. Persons become sick during their lifetimes. Teens experience bewilderment and lack of direction and identity. Parents and grandparents grow old, get sick, and die. Families with the complementary power of male and female can serve such redeeming purpose.

In the ethical system we are proposing, moral imperatives affirm the reciprocity of suffering and care effecting redemption. The dictates of biology and theology—indeed, of all vectors—produce not the radical differentiation and polarity of male and female but an efficacious complementarity in the life drama of burden bearing. Embryologists show us that, except for genetic encoding on the sex chromosome, the original embryonic being is an undifferentiated male/female. Then occurs the subtle transformation: tissues unfold with slight difference; different hormonal forces click in or remain dormant, exquisitely creating male or female in the proper populational balance. Sometimes an ambiguous birth requires a decision—

shall it be a boy or girl? Then the surgical and medicinal therapies confirm that arbitrary choice, and we are reminded of the biologic affinity of male and female. Theology also follows this wisdom: "male and female created he them."

Today we live in a world estranged from its natural and normative origins. Today, in obedience to the value of assumed suffering for another, we must argue against chauvinism and radical feminism and rather affirm this male/female reciprocity. For the sake of extraordinary anguish facing women in our future, this imperative is urgent.

We have entered a new world of biotechnology where it may become possible for men not only to share with women the figurative burden of childrearing, which indeed they should, but also the literal burden of childbearing. New developments in Australia and at other fertility/gestation laboratories are experimenting with ectopic pregnancies of various sorts, not excluding body cavities in the male torso. This new world will force us to affirm what particular gender roles, if any, we choose to affirm. It may also increase our sympathetic capacity.

Our deepest traditions of male-female reciprocity in the face of suffering and the belief that this contributes to edification and redemption of life should lead us to affirm that man and woman not be torn asunder. Persons are made and meant to be together. Biologic wisdom and all cognate wisdom points in this direction.

One of the clearest reminders of this "natural right" is the modern experience with divorce. In America, the culture of divorce in one generation is rapidly creating a culture of noncommitment in the next. Making a life together work appears to involve so much agony and the final denouement brings so much viciousness that young people are now testing whether the benefits of marriage can perhaps be gained through simple uncomplicated "relationships." This desire to settle life back at levels of precommitment and unhardship is part of a more general malaise of our time involving being together that is not fully human.

A second major area of ethical concern involving love and marriage has to do with the transience and technicality of relationships. Casual sexuality has replaced both the intense romantic and sanctified versions of an earlier era. As sex has become easy and omniavailable, it has lost its erotic and mystical quality. Becoming, as it has, more and more a technology (think of the massive literature and film on sexual technique), it has sunk more into the realm of apathy and away from the realm of passion. The violence of some

sex cultism and the virulence of pornography, by their very eruption, give further evidence that we are involved in very serious violation of a natural and sublime good.

Friendship is being there in better and in worse, in sickness and
in health. Knowing our propensity to want to escape when trouble
comes, our liturgical vows have stressed this constancy. The yearning to be rid of any pain and distress is ultimately a death longing.
The perfectly placid state is the state of nonbeing. Unless we can
reestablish a higher vision, a common purpose, or more likely a revelation, our increasing apathy will become more and more a death
journey. The cosmos and *oikos*, our world and habitat, penetrate
through to us in revelatory power through both the apocalyptic and
naturalistic (biologic) veils, disclosing a way of being and being together that both honors those imperatives that stand over against us
and satisfies our innermost desire.

The ethic of being alone or being together, of joining or split-
ting, is rigorous in the traditions of creation, apocalypse, and new
creation such as Judaism and Christianity. "It is not good that the
man should be alone. . . . He [made] a woman, and brought her unto
the man. . . . Therefore shall a man leave his father and mother, and
shall cleave unto his wife: and they shall be one flesh. . . . What
therefore God hath joined together, let not man put asunder. . . . I
am come to set a man at variance against his father" (Gen. 2:18, 22,
24; Matt. 19:61; 10:35).

This composite biblical teaching portrays a terrifying and wonderful world into which creatures who were receptors of the divine
image were placed. They were related together for a purpose, and
the relation was never to supersede the purpose. They were put
there as coworkers in a venture that involved suffering, death, and
transfiguration. God did not, as the Romantics supposed, botch up
the creation with a second effort because he was infuriated. He released a potential into this world that could be realized only
through freedom, striving, and then accomplishment. While these
reflections are vastly removed from a static ecological or even vibrant biologic sensibility about human partnership, they do resonate with those primal norms and bring them into proper relief.

The ordinary norm of sexual being together is clarified by considering several extraordinary modes of expression of sexual being
and sexual behavior. Celibacy, homosexuality, premarital sexuality,
and adultery—themes which have preoccupied the moral literature
across the millennia—further illustrate the position that the ethical
system we are proposing will support. Such evaluation will also

continue setting the building blocks of a comprehensive natality ethic.

Celibacy is a sign of hope for a world that may be living at the end of time. It can serve as an example to chaste living within the more dominant modes of sexual being. It is a life-style that may allow greater intensity of devotion. Celibacy, as priests and sisters are instructed, is an act of mortification, representation, and glorification—a fully human and a fully sexual commitment. It is not, however, a norm, and periods which have sought to establish celibacy as normative or a higher way have been misguided. Celibacy (from the point of view of sexual being) and childlessness (from the point of view of procreativity) are special callings which witness to the transience of life, the possibility that this world is passing away, and the sheer preeminence of the reality of God and eternity.

While there is absolutely no relinquishing of the richness of human sexuality and conviviality in the single life, and while that life may be populationally and apocalyptically adaptive, it remains a symbol of a cleft, an incompleteness, a pain at the heart of the cosmos. In a world where the toil of life, disease, war, and greater genetic fragility disproportionately diminish the male population so that there is an excess of females, the moral imperative requires not only that we receive with gratitude the contributions of single and widowed women but that we attend them with special care, since they bear in their body the fact that the world is not yet ready or whole.

Homosexuality, another mode of sexual being, has been thrown into profound confusion during the AIDS pandemic. Homosexuality and sterility intensify in congested bell-jar fly populations and, we might extrapolate, in crowded cities. We know that genetic and biochemical factors predispose persons to the condition. Early socialization where the male/female identity formation is confused seems to play a part. Certain environments such as boarding schools, navy ships, and monasteries may be conducive to the behavior. All persons, as we have noted, are in some rudimentary sense bisexual, and the fact that this is a labile characteristic allows us to move in either or both directions.

That perhaps 5 to 15 percent of our society may be homosexual is no reason for castigation or homophobia. This too is an exceptional state of sexual being, one that expresses breakage in the structure of the life-world and the cosmos itself. It is not a matter of blame or alarm. As is so often the case, nature provokes compensation where there is pain, so that an exceptional creativity has been offered the world from the gay and lesbian community. Again, the moral system which we have proposed would not make homosexuality normative or even position it as an equally valid alternative life-style. It is a state of being that we must abide graciously because the world is broken apart in pain and is not yet what it is meant to be.

The AIDS crisis is giving new energy to the vicious response of punishment and scapegoating, which, of course, is a shallow understanding of what has gone wrong in the world. The fundamentalist and neopuritan response to AIDS is nothing more than the snake's release of deeper venom. Three children who contracted AIDS through blood transfusions were refused admission to church and school, then fire-branded and run out of town in Arcadia, Florida. This unconscionable malevolence against innocence increases the crucifixion of the world. It may well be that countless babies will die of AIDS along with a sizable portion of the homosexual community in America, all the while the larger gay community is being harassed, quarantined (even more than it now is in urban ghettos), even killed, all as vicarious victims sacrificed to a furious world. Yet even this cleansing, this crucifixion, like the Civil War that Lincoln chronicled in his Second Inaugural Address, must needs come in order that redemption be wrought and righteousness be established.

Premarital sexual activity has greatly diminished in recent years. The may be due to the fear of AIDS and not some moral renewal, but it may portend some serious self-examination. Why forgo sexual relations until marriage, young people ask? Parents trying to protect their children from grief say things like: "The Bible forbids it"; "Your marriage won't be as pure and rewarding"; "You'll catch VD"; or "You'll get into the wrong crowd." Young people make counterarguments on each point: "Religion tells me to find authentic relationships"; "It will give me experience and cut down the divorce rate if we've checked each other out"; and "It's better to live now with one person than to play around." Our moral system simply asks, Does it heal and build or wound and hurt?

Adultery, or extramarital sex, is less difficult to condone and easier within this moral system to proscribe. Most often extramarital sex becomes a wretched process of compounding pain and amplifying suffering for all persons involved. It traverses the procreative, unitive, and protective values of human sexuality. While some Freudians might see the practice as psychically liberating, broader social and historic wisdom finds it disruptive. Finally, sex divorced from love and fidelity negates eternal value, confuting theological and eschatological bearings.

An ethic of sympathy will, in the end, stand by those who falter and fall. Those who break down and journey into far countries often touch the redemptive quick of reality, turn around, and discover true moral goodness, refreshingly vibrant when compared to drab conventionalism.

We have explored the moral meanings of being sexual and being together and, at the same time, have cast some light on the biologic component of ethics. This capacity in our moral soul for affection and shame, closely related to what the Greeks called conscience (suneidēsis), is our guide through decisions in this realm of experience. Now we become aware that we are more than an animal soul. We are rational and spiritual souls. These successive levels yield additional moral dimensions. To these we now turn.

4 Psychic Ethics of Autism and Attachment:

BEING WITH CHILD

The easiest way to judge a culture is how it treats its pregnant women.
Howard Haggard, *Devils, Drugs, and Doctors*

　　As W. H. Auden was viewing paintings in an exhibition, he stopped to reflect on Breughel's "Icarus." In this work the artist depicts a high-cliffed land crag overlooking a seascape—an eerie atmosphere created by a placid nature scene of a farmer plowing and a ship sailing, juxtaposed against the apocalyptic insert of a boy falling to his death. Our moral life is shaped by such serenity and surprise, prompting attitudes of apathy and passion and behavioral dialectics of autism and attachment. Confronted by suffering, we can be blind and oblivious or seeing and concerned. This great drama of detachment or engagement takes place in the feeling soul,

51

the psyche. The ultimate act of attachment, of giving oneself to another, is to be linked to a new life within one's body. The moral issue of being with child thus serves us well as a window to look at the nature of psychic ethics and the contribution of this school to a comprehensive ethical system.

We begin with the case history of a young African couple who was being cared for in an OB clinic. Sonography showed that the mother was carrying triplets. In accord with standard medical care in such cases, cesarean-section delivery was proposed. The family objected. They wrote a letter which all family members signed, claiming that the "natural" delivery of these babies was necessary for the political salvation of their African homeland. They also claimed that the deity they worshiped, the god of Abraham and Pascal, also required natural birth. Since the mother's life and those of the babies were thought to be threatened, the hospital decided to seek a court order for surgery. The order was given by reason of the rather bizarre grounds for the objection and the prevalent medical opinion that C section was indicated. The triplets were delivered well, and the mother recovered nicely. Shortly after the babies were born, the father committed suicide.

This agonizing case illustrates many of the ethical issues that present themselves in contemporary perinatal medicine. Contrasting views of the proper ways to give birth were present. The "natural" view was seen to be in conflict with the "scientific" medical view. The meaning of rights—of mother, family, the babies—was raised. The interests of the society were expressed through the court. Psychologically and culturally driven values and beliefs were found to be in conflict with legal and clinical conventions.

From ecology to eschatology all of the aspects of ethics we have found to be pertinent are expressed in this case. The story sets before us the potential for salutary resolution or tragedy, the transacting arch of meaning that we find spreading its way across all human experience. In retrospect, the case affirms one of our cardinal ethical axioms: an action is right as it ameliorates suffering and wrong as it amplifies it.

THE MORAL STATUS OF BEING WITH CHILD

I have argued that the ontology of being male and female imbues normative quality as does the unity of a man and woman. This is true not only because of the biologic givens of life which convey nature and purpose but also because of the other spheres of value which inform and are in turn informed by the biologic. Now we go a step further. What of the unique moral status entailed when a woman and, in a very important sense, both a man and a woman are "with child"? When we claim that this ontological status implies value, we mean it in two senses. We possess this *good* status because it has been given and we have received it from the author of life. We speak of being the "heirs" of the "grace of life." In another sense, the dyad (man and woman, husband and wife together) and the triad (mother, father, and child) present a further claim, a demand for acknowledgement, respect, and help. Value, in this sense, is both inherent and imputed.

Let us look at the natural and supernal grounding of this new status of being which is intrinsically valuable. The experience of being with child is said to have both a mundane and a mysterious quality. On the one hand, a new burden of life has sprung up within the life-support system of another. The woman is no longer alone. Morning sickness presages the numerous imcompatibilities and griefs that are inevitable when any two persons are bound together. Delight at hearing the heartbeats or feeling the kicking of tiny feet symbolize that lifelong experience of taking pleasure in the accomplishments of another throughout burdens and blessings.

There is also mysterious convivality in this elaboration of being. Margaret Mead, observing the primal natural experience of women with child in numerous field studies, found a quality of ecstasy in being "on the way" to some unknown state, of being an intimate part of something greater than oneself. "Each woman, knowing she is pregnant and knowing whose child she is carrying, must still be prepared, like her most primitive forebears, to cherish a being not yet known to her. And each woman is still left to ponder the mystery in her heart."[1]

The natural vindication of the state of being with child as a position of value is seen in the respect now given to the woman. The fellowship of "the sisters," the circle of supporting friends, now swings into action. Even if it is just a baby shower or some token gesture from one's otherwise unavailable working friends, the meaning is clear: Something special is happening to you, and we are with you. Most societies also accord certain privileges to "one great with child." Whether it is founded in an analogy of the "sick role" and a conferred patient status or in the sociologically derived maternity leave, the broader community, though not intimately involved, acknowledges a special condition deserving recognition and respect.

But in circumstances of general hostility—for instance, in war or street violence—special treatment is rarely afforded pregnant women. Though Nazi policy was opposed to abortion among its own people, the practice was condoned, even coerced, on "parasite" populations. Beyond this, esteem was contradicted by violence toward those who were with child and their offspring. "An Austrian midwife was in charge of drowning prisoners' [French Jews and resisters'] newborn babies in buckets of water. She told Genevieve de Gaulle that it took 20 to 30 minutes to drown them, such was their lung capacity. 'I was deported for practicing abortions,' the midwife said, 'and now I'm drowning babies.' "[2] In more customary circumstances, however, it would seem that something like a natural respect with a willingness to protect and help is offered to the woman known to be or seen to be with child.

The strongest evidence for the establishment of a natural value for the woman with child is the antipathy toward interrupting pregnancy that appears in all cultures throughout the ages. Whether it be the harsh laws of the Assyrian Empire in the second millennium B.C., where the aborting mother was impaled on a stake, or the policies of modern secular societies, where abortion is accepted (e.g. Japan), a mood of sadness, disappointment, and anger is found when a woman with child is undone without being delivered.

Perhaps the strongest affirmations of the dignity, high worth, and, therefore, the protectability and honor due the woman with child do not come from natural dignity but from the idea of alien dignity. Here the emphasis is on value that is bestowed from beyond rather than some inherent natural value. Two directions of alien dignity are found in the moral tradition. In the first, conception itself is viewed as the action of some external force using the instrumentality of the particular man and woman. Anchored in primitive moral consciousness where spirits, benign and malign, were the causal agents of all events, this view saw the human actors as passive in the miracle of conceiving life. This view does not enjoy great currency today as we exert more control over the process of conception. But since infertility research and conception technology have yet to explain fully or completely master the moment of conception, something of a creative miracle remains in the inception of life.

The other view of being with child that grounds human value more firmly holds that the mystery and miracle of this precious status is conveyed in the very natural grace of a man and woman, the binding act of love and the liberation of life through that blending of lives and mingling of flesh. "That which we beget," writes Oliver O'Donovan, "is like ourselves." Yet, "we do not determine what our offspring is, except by ourselves being that very thing which our offspring is to become, that which we beget can be, and should be, our companion . . . all human beings begotten of other human beings are, at the same time, made by God."[3] The modern transformation of human procreation into a technical operation, where begetting is reconceived as making, sometimes sweeps aside any such understanding as sentimental or fantastic. Yet reverence for life does linger on in the human soul and in the "common faith." It finds expression as the ground of inestimable value by which we commit ourselves to the survival and enhancement of the new being of life within life. The woman is now joined to this new life in common vitality, and the family and community are united with them in compassion. The virtue that undergirds and safeguards "being with child," this new ontology of value, springs from human psychology—the realm of consciousness, feeling, conscience, and will. Part of this transformation of soul enables a woman to become a mother.

MAMA

The genius of being a mother, that which provides the moral basis of mother with child or madonna and child, is the extraordinary generosity, partially supplied by instinct—and, one might surmise, this often against one's better judgment. This quality of giving oneself over to a life-sustaining symbiosis, giving up one's career and other pursuits of self-interest—indeed, giving of oneself as if the baby were oneself and then giving over (dramatically in birth and slowly across life) this bond of flesh and blood, tearing this other one away from one's self in the rupture of birth and the departure through growth—this is the unique and life-giving virtue of the woman.

In this primal unity of mother and child, ample provision is given for nurture, first through umbilical sustenance, and then, at birth, through the breast and the total embrace of care. This ample provision responds to acute need and helplessness in the offspring. In this primal unification, suffering is perfectly absorbed into help, and we are in a sense lifted beyond good and evil in a perfectly serene moral state. Erich Neumann writes:

With the emergence of the fully-fledged ego, the paradisal situation is abolished; the infantile condition in which life was regulated by something ampler and more embracing, is at an end, and with it the natural dependence on that ample embrace. We may think of this paradisal situation in terms of religion, and say that everything was controlled by God; or we may formulate it ethically, and say that everything was still good and that evil had not yet come into the world. Other myths dwell on the "effortlessness" of the Golden Age, when nature was bountiful, and toil, suffering and pain did not exist; others stress the "everlastingness" of the Golden Age, the deathlessness of such an existence.[4]

Fetal bliss is offered by the shield of protection from external insult and of being alive too soon on one's own.

The outstanding characteristic of the higher mammals' development is the growth and maturation of the entire organization within the protection of the mother's body. All higher mammals are characterized by long periods of gestation, the duration of which is clearly related to the central nervous system's level of organization. Formed in the maternal uterus, and determined by the genetic plan specific to each species, is the entire apparatus of movement, the bodily posture appropriate to the species, and its typical instinctual organization, all of it tailored to an environment which is also genetically assigned to that species. Patterns of movement and behavior are formed in the mother's body, well-removed from later stimulus sources and yet oriented toward those subsequent stimuli, toward the future environment.[5]

The moral status of mother and child is established first by the woman's willingness to receive and create a new life. Without this willingness the world and the human story could not go on. Second, there is the readiness to provide the internal atmosphere for life sustenance without which that life could not thrive and come into full being. The continuity of the human story and the shielding from danger of a life incapable of self-protection and self-sustenance are two of the cardinal values of mother and child.

Recent research on maternal-child health is also showing that this value is not only ontic, it is operational. Although we find an awesome resilience and invulnerability in the conceived child, the value of continued existence through gestation and birth of a baby is not ensured just by the state of pregnancy. We now know that mothercraft, the art and care of being a mother, is essential for healthy gestation and safe delivery.[6] We also know that an awesome dependence on the mother, abject dependence for vitality and wellness, is found in the fetus. Not only do inadequate nutrition, substance abuse, over- and underweight, and ill-fitness leave their mark on the fetus, far subtler factors, such as maternal depression, can suppress the birth weight and general wellness of the baby.[7] Lives literally are tethered together in a life-and-death drama. The child also serves a redeeming moral function for the mother; it releases her from the sin of narcissism so pervasive and ruthless in the male and even the female of the species. Now love is directed beyond oneself.

When we use the words *mother, mama, muter, mater,* and all the other cognates in the languages of the world, we use an archetypal image. *Mother* represents the energy from which we came and the source to which we return. We use images and symbols such as heaven, earth, the woods, the seas, the fields, gardens, springs, flowers, the rose—all conveying vital origins, protection from harm, safe return. The ubiquitous representation of madonna and child in all cultures, in all historical periods, represents an eternal image—life giving, sheltering, enfolding from harm and danger.[8] Rather than this being Jungian fantasy, it is the persistent way human language refers to the undeniable moral significance of mother and mother/child.

In the situation of being with child, the father's role is to uphold his wife, as the wife's role is to educate her husband. He must try to provide for the family so that she is free to carry the baby in peace, free from anxiety. He must also assure the mother of the dignity and inestimable worth of the travail she has entered and will endure. This is especially needed in a world which no longer cherishes children or honors mothers with child. In a world that prizes career advancement and entrepreneurial achievement, a woman often wonders why she should bother with being a mother. Finally, father must safeguard the child, perhaps even in exceptional circumstances, against the wishes of mother, offering that unique driving-out yet upholding support.

The discussion of the morale of a mother and father now with child and the distinctive moral emphasis that each brings to the triadic relation also provides insight into the psychic structure of ethics. Referring to mother and father in a metaphoric sense and noting role-specific attributes raises the possibility that there is a corresponding dialectic in the moral soul. If the community is the individual writ large, perhaps the individual is the community writ small. When we study human nature in relationships, we see that overcaring attachment and overbearing authority are the two radical poles of danger framing a spectrum of possibility of psychic moral responses.

THE PSYCHIC COMPONENT OF ETHICS

Toward the one pole, autism is complete withdrawal from the external pain of life, since the inner pain is already so great. Apathy is the suppression of feeling, anxiety about getting hurt. Attraction is the rudimentary impulse of being drawn near to another. Attachment is joining oneself to another or another to oneself out of loyalty, need, or duty. Affection is the willingness to risk hurt for the sheer delight of contact with another.

When we speak of the psychic component of ethics, we find ourselves poised between the biologic and philosophical realms. When we probe the feeling and emotion of affection, for example, we have come to a level above animal attraction and appetite, yet below the rational philosophy of Stoic *apatheia* or Epicurean *ataraxia* (tranquility). In psychic ethics, we are dealing with four dimensions of the human spirit: consciousness, feelings, conscience, and will. Being with child, the primary extension of care outside of the self and beyond the male-female bond, calls into play these fundamental levels of psychic ethics.

The animation whereby persons relate—in this case, where two parents relate to a developing child—gathers together these four dimensions of the human spirit, creates a single animus, and forms a crucial dimension of ethics. All human relations are occasions for responsibility. They are also experiences which build up "living strengths"—virtues which are fashioned in the human race across the span of evolution and in individuals during their development.

A number of critical moral insights emerge from the psychic domain. *Consciousness* itself is of enormous moral import. It is the closest attribute to life itself. Though one who is unconscious is still alive, permanent unconsciousness, irretrievable coma, or persistent vegetative states signal that life is gone and death is at hand. Consciousness contributes to ethics not only as we imbue the state of being with value, but as it becomes the foundation of all modes of perception and awareness. Consciousness itself, it can be argued, is the value of life.

Feelings are a primary focus of the moral life in its psychic dimension. Impulses ranging from kindness and pity to rage, shame, and guilt all play vital roles in the moral life. The range of emotions that enrich our being should be welcomed, be expressed not repressed, and be honored as legitimate sources of virtue and authority. The anatomy of feelings has been drawn by many writers, Willard Gaylin's being one of the most insightful.[9] Emotions play a crucial role in the moral system we have proposed because suffering itself, a theme in our leitmotif, is posited upon the biologic axis of pain and pleasure and upon the psychological axis of sadness and happiness. In our rudimentary sense, irritation becomes pain which, when added to illness, becomes physical suffering. Suffering compounded with moral significance becomes evil. Just as there are distinctions to be made between natural and moral evil, so distinctions must be made between physical and metaphysical suffering. In any case, the pathetic soul, the feeling faculty of the moral soul, is the mediator of this discernment. In one sense, suffering is an evaluation of what is happening. Though it is provoked by crude stimulus-response and rooted in even more refined feelings and antipathies, suffering is primarily a value.

To return to the clinical example of this chapter, pregnancy and childbirth is normally not considered an illness or an occasion of suffering. Even pain and anesthesia in childbirth has been a controversial theme. In the nineteenth century, debates raged as to whether analgesia or anesthesia was proper for childbirth pain. Perhaps this was the paradise fall that had to be allowed to run its course for the edification of one's soul. A great debate raged about the thresholds of pain and how this varied by gender, race, temperament, age, and social condition.[10]

In the twentieth century, a strange polarization of birth practice has developed, even in the advanced technological world. On the one hand, pregnancy and birth have been drawn more and more under the reach of technology and pharmacology. Sophisticated monitoring, technological visualization, refined anesthetics, and frequent cesarean-section birth (now approximately 25 percent in America) have rendered birth a surgical and hospital event. At the same time, beginning in the 1950s, two French methods of childbirth—Lamaze and LeBoyer—have given expression to a massive movement in the direction of natural childbirth, home birth, birth free from clinical, surgical, and pharmacological trappings. The dialectics of emotions, of feeling tones, of participatory involvement of the father, and of sympathetic pain sharing have all played a central role in this revolution.

Conscience can be seen as another feature of the psychic axis, a close cognate of emotionality. We speak of shame as a feeling of remorse usually associated with a sexual activity. We speak of guilt feelings. Many volumes have been devoted to exploring the nature and function of conscience. It was seen in classical literature as the force of the ideal standing over against the material. It was the ferocious wind of nemesis blowing back to haunt one after pride or misdeeds. In biblical thought, conscience was the searching light of the divine presence laying open the dark intentions and actions that we thought could be covered up. The New Testament speaks of conscience as a structure of the natural mind, which is enlivened by the Holy Spirit. In the eighteenth and nineteenth centuries, the conscience was often identified as the citadel and monitor of societal mores and conventions. From this history we receive Freud's rendition of conscience as superego—the stern reminder of parental dominance and societal ordinance. Today conscience has largely been subdued by autonomous will. We repudiate any qualms of conscience as subjective, relativistic, and repressive and brush them lightly aside. Renewal of the power of conscience will probably come as it is seen as a moral companion of knowledge itself—*conscientia*—a legitimate gauge of the feedback insight of the results of what we have done or what we are deciding to do. Conscience will come to have a postmorbid and a premonitory moral function. Conscience will also be renewed as it becomes a more precise instrument to assess the way in which our decisions and actions will hurt ourselves or others. Modern feedback cycles and cybernetic loops can enhance traditional conscience as a "what if" judgment on our contemplated actions.

Yet another element in the psychic capacity for knowing and doing good or evil is the *will*. The great volitionalist philosophers across the ages such as Luther, Erasmus, Fichte, Schelling, Hegel, and Schopenhauer would demand a separate treatise on the will. To some extent Freud himself accepted the philosophy of German idealism which subscribed to the reality of a blind subconscious natural will. Just as for Freud *Trieb* (poorly translated "instinct") is a primal force animating our perception and behavior, so the will is an awesome force profoundly shaping the moral life. In one sense, we speak of will as the dynamic that works through all dimensions of moral capacity. We speak of the "flesh being willing" and of "political will." For the purposes of this book, we will think of will not as an extraneous or independent force but as the working energy, the dynamic, to put moral power (virtue) into action from any direction. It is a crucial force because no matter how splendid the impulse, value, or vision, it is important and deprived of efficacy without intention and volition.

BEING WITH CHILD: ETHICAL ISSUES

In this light we shall now explore four ethical issues which involve a woman with child or a mother and father expecting a baby. The issues, selected from the many at this juncture of human natality, represent the kind of questions present more generally among the group. We first discuss pregnancy induction, with in-vitro fertilization as a case in point. Second, we consider the issue of maternal abuse of the fetus. Third, the question of coerced cesarean-section delivery is explored. Finally, we examine virtue in the various modes of childbirth. We begin this section with a statement of general ethical direction vis-à-vis "being with child."

Generativity, the desire to pass life on, is a virtue mingled with vice. We can conceive children for glory or for destruction (Isaiah 65). Woody Allen once quipped: "I don't want to achieve immortality through my works. I want to achieve immortality by not dying." The impulse for aggrandizement, ego perpetuation, and immortality can motivate persons to become pregnant and offer children to the world. The fruits of the womb can be nourishing or poisonous. The ignorant French farmer who kept having children only to kill them at birth said he did not know how to stop having babies and he could not feed them. This sad incident, reported in a Paris newspaper a few years ago, symbolizes the many children who are brought into the world so carelessly that they are doomed to tragic death. The scandal in the United States of postnatal death—death from deprivation and neglect in the first eighteen months of life—also reflects misbegotten generativity.

Being with child can offer a liberating of life, an opportunity for familial delight, an assumption of reciprocal obligation on behalf of the community, and a sacred trust. When a child is well conceived, born into a community that cares, all done in faithful vow before the giver of life, earth's pain is diminished and redemption flourishes. The foremost value in birth is the liberation of a new life. "Not every little being knocking on the door of life needs to be let in," Margaret Mead once said. She may have had a sound point in mind if she was attacking the vitalistic heresy where each germ cell and conceptus is seen as inviolable. Her point, though, is misleading. Each child on the way to being born *is* a gift to be cherished, unless some grievous consequence for that child or mother is threatened. The world is not a vast basin of potential beings all knocking on the door to get in. A life given miraculously to a ready mother and father is the provident and creative hand of God outstretched, a gift. Apart from any extrinsic or utilitarian value, the inestimable intrinsic value of a person more than justifies pregnancy and birth.

A second value is the realization of the covenant of family. Creation shrivels if composed only of individuals. Aggregates and the intimate aggregate and congregate of family draw forth the potential of personal beings and mutually shield and absorb the suffering that life inevitably brings. "The child is truly saved," said Luther in a baptismal sermon, "when the congregation means its baptism." In conception and birth a family expresses its duty to the community, and the society reciprocates with its commitments of nurture and protection. The terrible modern notion of disconnected nuclear families violates fundamental societal covenant. The family does not say to the society, "Here, he's yours—take care of him." Nor does the society say, "You're on your own—it's your kid." Family, extended family, and the broader community and society are heirs together and stewards henceforth of the grace of life.

Finally, receiving a child is a sacred trust. In all high religion, a child is the miraculous expression of God that life should continue and his will proceed. If new life arises from this divine ground, there is no longer room to think of pregnancy as an "accident," to speak of "one too many," to comment, "You're stuck with it," or to engage in any other of the disparagements of ingratitude. Certain provocative issues can now be viewed in the light of the broader moral system.

Pregnancy induction via a wide range of techniques is now available. Male and female fertility and fecundity can be enhanced through hormonal induction. Insemination via a donor or husband can be achieved artificially. Even when the channels of natural induction (fallopian-tube passage) are blocked, babies can be *made* by in-vitro fertilization and embryo transfer. These technologies surely serve the values of creating a new personal life and fulfilling parental desire. The difficulty in terms of our moral framework comes at the societal level. The tragic irony of millions of abortions, other millions of unwanted births, and thousands of poor children orphaned for want of adopting parents, all the while some thousands seek these exotic methods of pregnancy induction, is morally problematic.

A second ethical concern is the present haphazard enterprise of fertility manipulation and baby *making* as it takes the form of commercial business and industry. The Industrial Revolution, in the factory movement in England and Germany for example, sought to relieve toil (hard labor) and maximize pleasure (produce goods) but ended up frequently sacrificing both values. Mass production in baby making—whether it be the discarding of extra embryos in in-vitro fertilization or cases like multiple impregnation where five fetal sacs are started by stimulated ovulation and sperm induction and then three must be sacrificed in order that two survive—all this activity enlarges human waste and sacrifices the deep virtues of attachment, longing, identification, and nurturing care.

In-vitro fertilization has proven to be the most ethically provocative method of pregnancy induction. O'Donovan locates the moral problematic of IVF in the fact that medical practice is now shaped by the political ethos which he calls "the liberal revolution." In this era where personal freedom and release from suffering are made possible by technological enterprise, tragic reversal often occurs, and unforeseen anguish is created as much as supposed pain is relieved. This insult occurs both for physicians and patients.

> The medical practitioner finds himself an agent in the midst of a mass activity, and of course he can have no independence of action to speak of. If a certain medical technology has been developed, it is expected by society that he will facilitate his patients' access to it.... The paradox is that the community's goal is freedom; but such freedom clearly cannot include freedom of action which might frustrate communal action. It follows that we conceive our freedom passively, as a freedom not to suffer, not to be imposed upon.[11]

The ultimate freedom not to suffer is the freedom not to feel—the state of apathy or autism. Attachment, advocacy, and being for another involves risk and the potential for pain. Without suffering there can be no redemption. The quest for suffering-free procreation could someday lead to a Huxley's *Brave New World*, where all offspring are created by in-vitro decantation according to political needs—so many workers, scientists, warriors, and so forth. In that day, birth will be easy, for birth will no longer involve travail—or commitments—or persons.

A second moral comment on IVF relates to the apathy/attachment index in a tangential way. We shall devote a later chapter on genetic prediction to what we will call the epistemic ethics of knowledge and ignorance. In IVF we also have the crisis of unpredictability and the demand for certainty. In order to avert the suffering of the unknown, several embryos are implanted so that one has a modest chance of taking hold and flourishing. The experience of couples seeking IVF even in the major medical centers is still punctuated with disappointment and failure. Some IVF centers have yet to achieve a successful pregnancy. The moral imperative to achieve satisfaction and certainty should be sought only if it can continue to involve human participation. In O'Donovan's terms, the more we transpose human birthing into functional "making" and away from the human "begetting," the more we destroy the very good we seek in procreation. Taking the first theme from the Nicene Creed, O'Donovan argues that, just as Jesus was begotten not made and thereby was like God in every way so that human life could be transformed, so man and woman receive new life and give it to one like them, "bone of their bone and flesh of their flesh." In this way the passion and mystery of life goes on.

Another construal of the suffering/redemption connection that bears on IVF is found in the theological dynamics of providence and abandonment. Is one left to one's own devices, or does a divine scheme operate through all experience, delightful and discomforting? Trust in providence both allows the venture of risk and comforts adventurers that the future is not completely of their making. "To act well . . . requires faith in divine providence because one must hope (without the possibility of calculative proof) that what one has done will be used for the service of others rather than their hurt."[12]

The doctrine of providence, from its mighty origins in monotheistic and prophetic religion down through its elaboration in Christian experience and in the corroborative testimony of history and science, finds that even mistakes and malevolent acts are transformed through redemptive process into ongoing purpose. Here in defense of the practice of IVF we can refute the naysayers who hold that this conception technique should not be used because we could never guarantee long-range futures free of side effects. There might be genetic breakage or cellular trauma that would manifest itself only when the person thus conceived was forty years old, it was argued. Providence contends that acts done in human respect, in justice, and in piety will be fashioned to worthwhile purpose, even if they blunder. "Faith in the providence of God as the ruling power of history . . . acknowledges that there are limits to man's responsibility with regard to the future and that in 'acting well' we can contribute to the course of events a deed, which whatever may become of it . . . is fashioned rightly in response to the reality which actually confronts the agent."[13]

The possibility of accurately predicting harm and benefit to the fetus growing within a woman caused by her habits and behaviors now presents a new dimension of responsibility to a mother, a family, and the society. What is the nature of moral accountability now that harm can occur to the life within by such things as alcohol and cigarette abuse, heroin and other substance misuse, toxic exposure, even anxiety?

Many influences on the child within the mother can retard or impair development. Drugs such as Thalidomide and Bendictine warn us of the likelihood that many chemical compounds, perhaps even certain foods, insult the fetus to greater or lesser extent. New studies show that the health-food habits of the diet conscious—with diets, for example, of bean sprouts, skim milk, and broccoli—may indeed be harmful to the fetus. Calorie and iron deficiency likewise may take a toll. The effect of infections such as rubella virus is painfully remembered. Smoking may cause lower birth weight and actually increase newborn mortality. High alcohol consumption has been associated with mental retardation, growth failure, and birth defects. Furthermore, depression or more serious mental disturbances may transect even this most impressive protector, the placental barrier. Add to this the adverse effects of exposure to noxious and toxic influences in various workplaces, and we find ourselves in a situation of knowing many potential causes of harm and therefore confronted with new questions of personal and societal responsibility and liability.

Consider, for example, the issue of fetal alcohol syndrome as a case where a calculus of suffering comes to bear in making moral evaluations. Both the syndrome and the more general category of fetal alcohol effects are now clearly documented causes of fetal harm. Growth retardation and damage to the cardiovascular, neurological, and other major systems is firmly established.[14] Responsibility extends from the person to the family and the society. Options for preventive and ameliorative action include education, regulation, and incarceration. Who can say that it is better for all concerned for a woman not to work in the paint factory while she is pregnant? Perhaps being unemployed would bring greater suffering to her and the baby within her. The arguments about smoking and drinking run the same way. Is not the release from nervous anxiety thought to be afforded by narcotic effect preferable to the unabated life tension one feels without this crutch? On the other hand, the pain of deprivation borne for the sake of saving from suffering that helpless one to whom one is tethered in life's struggle is worthwhile. One sees here the tension between societally and systemically induced morbidity and that caused by careless personal actions.

Alcohol dependence often reflects family sickness. The family and often substitute family is also the best source of preventive and interventive care for alcoholism. When the individual is scapegoated to bear suffering vicariously in a family with a pathological burden, he or she often turns to alcohol abuse. Family healing can occur through various therapies, with Alcoholics Anonymous being the preeminent lifesaver because of its redemptive commitment. As the miners at Roaring Camp discovered in Bret Harte's tale "The Luck of Roaring Camp," the coming of a baby in the midst of a desperate scene can, in and of itself, transform the surrounding community.

Societies also seem to have harmful or healing effect when it comes to alcohol or other substance abuse. The Soviet Union and certain Amerindian communities seem to provoke alcohol abuse by brutalizing their citizens through constantly depressing conditions of life or destroying traditional outlets and patterns of support. In America, hard drug abuse now threatenes to destroy the whole fabric of society. The underlying cause ironically seems to be a tearing of the fabric of community support, interest in one another, provision of satisfying work, and a general conviviality that comes when people care for one another and bear one another's burdens. Again, in ameliorating the brutal force of substance abuse and in encouraging and supporting the inception of new life, the community plays a vital role by developing an élan vital which alone can restore a sense of bonding.

However, in order to safeguard the value of personal choice and initiative, the society should opt for methods of education to solve the problem of fetal abuse and wastage. When in the New Orleans parishes barefoot healers are sent to the shanties and tenements where pregnant girls live, and when these wise but poor women counsel these "children having children" about proper care for themselves and for the lives within them, we should not be surprised when all of the mishaps of pregnancy diminish, including premature births, and when the costs to society, including neonatal intensive care units, are greatly reduced. Regrettably we seemed to prefer to pay the high cost of NICUs, the tragedy of "preemie" births, and the greater tragedy of postnatal mortality when, starting in 1981, we proceeded to cut off funds for this social program. (See further discussion of this program in chapter 8.)

Should society resort to the harsher measures of regulation and incarceration to safeguard fetal lives which are developing within abusing mothers or families? The West German health-care system has a rigorous, somewhat authoritarian, program of maternal-child welfare called *Fürsorge*, their version of American services of care for families and children. This social service is undergirded by a body of regulatory statutes traditionally based on child-abuse law which is now being extended to cover fetal abuse. Regulation fits ethical response to the exceptional value of protecting women bearing children, especially if it is nurturing and helpful regulation that provides maternal grants, work leaves, free services, and voluntary care programs, and not just harsh rules devoid of aid. The most controversial issue of mother-and-child ethics today concerns the freedom-constraining power of the state. Should pregnant women who threaten the lives of their offspring be held against their will, have their behaviors coercively modified, and for all practical purposes be incarcerated so that their babies are well born? Two cases highlight this moral quandary.

A woman who was pregnant was detained by the Department of Children and Family Services (DCFS) in an attempt to restrain her heroin habit and the deleterious effect it might have on her fetus. The case was interesting for the fact that many experts argue that addictions are illnesses outside of the volition control of the victims and, indeed, do require external help, perhaps even to the point of constraint.

The other case showed this point even more poignantly. The mother with child was diagnosed as a severe manic-depressive. She was being treated with medication involving significant amounts of mineral and metal substance which was known to be damaging to the fetus. Two moral questions emerged. Was a mentally ill woman fit to be a mother? Should the fetus be aborted by a medically requested court order? This decision was pondered at the same time that a Texas mother was requesting a court-ordered abortion for her twelve-year-old daughter, who wanted to keep her baby. The political mood in the country at the time was prolife.

In the case of the manic mother, an abortion order was not sought, and the pregnancy continued. The baby was delivered and taken home. During the first winter of the baby's life, the child was found frozen stiff on the back porch of her apartment, where it had been left during a frigid Chicago night. Like the case of the African family with triplets and the father's suicide after a coerced cesarean delivery, the aftermath of this case called into question the decision not to abort. In the triplet case autonomy was overridden in order to prevent presumably likely suffering and death and ended up causing suffering and death. In the manic-depressive case autonomy was honored but suffering and death ensued, albeit only harder and later than it would have with the abortion. Was redemption served in either case? Were the psychodynamic ethics of autism or attachment followed?

One virtue of the ethical system under consideration is its pluridimensionality. Life is sacred when seen from a theological and eschatological viewpoint. That personal abilities must be considered we know on psychic and biologic grounds. The enveloping social, political, and legal climate not only reflects other dimensions of value but itself creates value. Throughout all, the redemptive motif allows us to see purpose in suffering, death, and transfiguration. It prompts us to preserve persons from harm and to proffer help. Such an ethic encourages us to live boldly and gratefully in a world full of risk and shrouded in the unknown. Men and women should receive the gift of new life with a sense of awe-filled mystery and responsible stewardship. We do not want to create further a world where parents are afraid of begetting children. Now that the increasing range of risks (even highly improbable risks) is being made known, one wonders why any woman would be willing to carry and mother a child. To bear a child requires that one forgo or, at least, detain or interrupt one's career. It requires loving someone into life against a world that not only fails to honor and remunerate the act but actually, in some grotesque ways, holds a woman with child in contempt or blame. Only a moral vision at once deeper and higher than mere calculating pragmatism, a vision accompanied by committed burden sharing by others, only such a sacrificial new day of cohumanity can serve us from a future of technological anomie.

A clinical ethical issue related to maternal restraint is that of *coerced cesarean-section delivery*. Stimulated by the triplet case mentioned at the opening of this chapter, a group of obstetricians published an important study on enforced C-section deliveries. The cases illuminate another important field of concerns in natality ethics where the values of a society—codified in laws and policies and court casuistry—interacts with scientific (rational) values about "good" medical practice and personal and familial values of freedom. The findings of this study are surprising.

> In a national survey, we investigated the scope and circumstances of court-ordered obstetrical procedures in cases in which the women had refused therapy deemed necessary for the fetus. Court orders have been obtained for . . . caesarean sections, intrauterine transfusions and hospital detentions . . . the court orders were obtained in 86 percent of cases [petitioned]. . . . 81 percent of the women were black, Asian, or Hispanic, 44 percent were unmarried. . . . And the women were treated in teaching-hospital clinic or were receiving public assistance.[15]

The survey of physican attitudes and values about overriding the objections of mothers and families showed divided opinion. About half of those questioned felt that the prospective well-being and survival of the fetus merited intervention. Another half felt that these values of amelioration and salvation of babies did not merit violating a woman's autonomy and subjecting her to harm.

Should a woman be forced to safeguard her fetus even if it involves some risk to herself? Should parents be allowed to withdraw attachment from children they have conceived? In one remarkable case a court pressed on a mother the duty to care for and pay for care of her teenage daughter's baby. The wild confusion of natality ethics is evidence when we set this case alongside the case of the grandmother in South Africa giving birth via IVF to her own daughter's triplets.

The morality derived from human psychology that we have explored in this chapter makes clear that inner strength (virtue) is necessary to ethical awareness and assumption of responsibility. It is very hard to argue that our society has sufficiently imbued teenage girls from indigent ethnic backgrounds with the kind of experience and support that would justify the expectation of mature responsibility. Taking over for them now the decisions about obstetric care—detaining them in hospital, forcing cesarean delivery—then abandoning them to care unassisted for misconceived and misdelivered babies is an unconscionable amplification for suffering. The study concludes:

Such developments [more assumption of prerogatives by the state overriding patient objection] could . . . prove to be counter productive to public policy goals for maternal and infant health. If court-ordered obstetrical procedures become more common, the public image of hospitals may be adversely affected and women may choose to deliver elsewhere [perhaps a good idea!]. The groups that are most in need of prenatal care may be driven away from it . . . and [if home birth replaces hospital birth] more harm than good would result.[16]

Mention of home birth brings us to consider a final issue of maternal-child care—the various *modalities of birth*. A wide range of more natural birth modalities is epitomized by the psychoprophylactic mode of childbirth free from pain, popularly known as Lamaze. Developed across the years at the Maternité in Paris, the method is now widely practiced around the world. We offer brief praise for it as we close this chapter on women with child because of its unique philosophy about pain and delivery. Lamaze also exemplifies a moral psychology of involvement when one is tempted by the fear of birthing travail to disengage from the experience.

If there is value in bringing children into the world and virtue, therefore, in the status "being with child," it follows that birth should be transacted in a way to optimize the bond of affection between mother and child and soften her resistance to the labor. Need pregnancy and childbirth be viewed as it has through the ages—as a curse? Lamaze writes: "For millennia a curse has hung over mankind. Childbirth and pain appeared wedded forever in close and mutually dependant bondage. No other fate seemed imaginable. So women, fearful and resigned, passively consented to suffer the most exalting act in her life."[17]

Man's toil and women's travail—the labor of them both—should not be seen as punishment or curse. The experience of childbirth can be viewed as a sacrifice of joy that brings renewal of life. Lamaze projects back from the twentieth century largely masculine images of pain and anguish. The experience of birth is universal, natural, and immemorial, not cataclysmic or severe, as nineteenth-century mechanists thought, an anguish to obliterate and a problem to fix. The whole idea that pregnancy is a disease is the extrapolate of Victorian and modern technology and anesthetic philosophy. Beginning in the early modern era, medicine began to offer its fateful promise to prevent pain and tragedy. Twilight sleep and other anesthetics rendered women unaware of the entire birth process. Birth was removed to hospitals away from homes, to obstetricians away from midwives, from awareness to anesthesia, all in the illusory quest to alleviate a curse. New suffering followed in the wake of the conquest. Puerperal fever in septic hospitals made childbirth much more life threatening to mother and baby than it ever was at home. Obstetrics was as iatrogenic a specialty as bloodletting. Drugs did and still do cause birth injury.

Only now is our philosophy of pain and our moral psychology about suffering beginning to shift, so that we can view birth anguish in a different, more constructive light. Part of the enlightenment is that, thanks to Lamaze and the earlier pioneer in natural birth, Grantly Dick-Read, we are beginning to see pain in a more wholistic context.

Lamaze learned his theory and methods from the Russian stimulus-response psychologists in the Pavlovian tradition. Like the Cartesians of France and the Puritans of England three centuries later, the Pavlovians had the genius of being simultaneously mechanical and metaphysical thinkers. Pain was analyzed in its objectivity and subjectivity because, like the particle-and-wave theory of light, explanation and understanding could be achieved only by complementarity. The objective side of pain, whether it be from burn, bump, hot, cold, sting, prick, or scrape, was an unconditioned stimulus response signaled by pain pathways into the brain cortex, where, after complex interactions with subjective elements of interpretation, it was perceived as pain. Lamaze concludes: "Pain is neither a simple mechanical process nor a mysterious 'psyche' one. . . . Pain is an entity for too long looked upon as made up of two separate parts, a subjective and an objective one. Pain is a whole, and this unity of action of painful perception is an essential feature of the problem of pain in childbirth."[18]

The Lamaze method of birth, based on carefully practiced rote and rational responses in the midst of the anxiety, trauma, and urgency of labor, teaches us much about the ethics of natality in general and the particular ethics of childbirth. Should midwives be licensed to deliver babies? Should home births be discouraged, even proscribed? Many objective elements come into play as we make moral and policy decisions in this field. We need to temper our technological desires with appreciation of natural values. We need also to proceed with initiatives of thought and technique which enhance human values of procreation. We need to establish objective moral ordinance about birth so that mothers, fetuses, and babies are not abused. Paid maternity and paternity leaves should be made mandatory for employers. We should make provision for sustenance of mothers with child. Free access to optimal nutrition, housing, counselling, and moral support is the minimal obligation of any society that honors the lives entrusted to its care.

Exquisite sensitivity to the subjective sensibilities of individuals will also be required for sound ethics. The psychological dimension of ethics points up the centrality of personal moral response in any system. Individuals stand personally responsible to their God, their own conscience, and the truth and right as they understand it. At the same time, psychic ethics, like the vectors that preceded it and like those which follow, show us the necessary communality and conviviality of our life. Being with child is nature's wonderful reminder that we belong to each other.

5 Philosophical Ethics of Ending Life:

ABORTION

Watson: Holmes, you did not show that man great sympathy.

Holmes: He didn't come to me for sympathy.

Sir Arthur Conan Doyle, "The Case of the Dancing Men"

If conceiving and bearing a child is an ultimate act of attachment, the ultimate act of detachment is abortion. But as T. S. Eliot has written, "There is a time to care and a time not to care." Sherlock Holmes exemplifies the Victorian penchant for disinterested calculation, logic, and rational analysis of life's mysteries and moralities. There is a time for sympathy and a time for rationality. It seems best in the context of the ongoing inquiry of this book to join the most emotion-fraught issue of our time (abortion) with the most rational component of ethics (the philosophical).

While detachment of thought supposedly brings objectivity, affectional detachment inflicts pain on another. Well-being is that reciprocity of needing and helping that occurs when two lives meet. Whether it be in the literal act of abortion or the more common severance acts of alienation and isolation, tearing apart the sustaining ligatures of comfort and undergirding expose the one cut off to vulnerability, harm, and death. To abort any ongoing story of life bonded to life is a moral atrocity. Condemnation and damnation literally mean to be cut off from life sustenance and support.

Strong words? Yes! Yet, beyond this truth is an even deeper truth. Originally and ultimately everyone stands alone. Before and after incorporation everyone is cut off. We emerge from nothing into birth and life. We descend toward nothing in disease, deterioration, and death. Our being together with others is a momentary grace between the deeper mystery of what lies before and after. Part of our ethical life is ascetic, achieved as we are apart and alone. Another part plays itself out as we are incorporated, joined together. In some way the cosmic and apocalyptic dimensions of ethical reality at one end of the spectrum and the theological and eschatological dimensions at the other end are symbols we use to convey this existential aspect of responsibility. We stand alone not against the void but against God, the ground and culmination of being.

The middle spectrum of ties and bonds to which we now turn signifies convivial responsibility. Here biologic, psychic, historical, and social contexts give shape to values. The two moral powers that we now explore—the philosophical, and the epistemic—are, in one sense, abstractions over the entire system. Our total scheme can be seen as an all-embracing moral philosophy.

Abortion arises as one of the most perplexing concerns to trouble the human soul at the bridge point where that terrible and wonderful aloneness becomes togetherness. In the abortion controversy we talk about the preexistent being in the divine wisdom and about the detached value of the human fetus. "Before you were fashioned in the womb, I knew you." "It's a tissue of my body." In the modern age of sensibility toward suffering and of assigning independent value to each unique being, we talk of an autonomous destiny or the "potential life" of a fetus. Here we are affirming some ontological status apart from incorporation into a woman. It then appears as if ethical justice requires that we deal with a fetus in its own right. At the same time, since fetal protection and enhancement, on the one hand, and abortion, on the other, are of necessity issues where two or more lives are inextricably intertwined, we cannot talk of unilateral responsibility.

THE ABORTION CRISIS: PAIN IN THE FETUS

Our primary moral responsibility is to receive and nurture life and to not inflict suffering. We have noted the extent to which society is willing to go to enhance the health of a developing human being (fetal therapy and the like). We continue to struggle with the unresolved question of ethics in abortion policy. In this vein, many argue that the first issue to explore in the abortion debate is the inflicting of pain on a fetus. Surprisingly, this concern is shared by those who condone and those who oppose abortion. The former group feel that finding the least painful mode of abortion would be a merciful action as the widespread practice continues. Those who oppose abortion use the "pain infliction" argument as a building block in establishing their position.

The most widely practiced means of abortion today are curettage (a euphemism for cutting apart), suction and curettage, the saline contamination of the amniotic bath, and the injection of prostaglandins. In early pregnancy (where pain thresholds may be different than in later development), a sharp knife is used to kill the unborn child. In suction curretage, a vacuum pump sucks up the unborn child by bits and pieces and a knife severs the remaining parts. In the second trimester or later, a hypertonic saline solution is injected into the amniotic fluid. That the salt poisons and scalds the fetus is evidenced when the fetus is delivered covered with burns as if it had been soaked in acid. Prostaglandins enter the fetal circulation and disrupt cardiac function so that the fetus dies either in or ex utero. John Noonan reflects on the pain and suffering of these procedures.

> Are these experiences painful? The application of a sharp knife to the skin and vital tissue of the fetus cannot but be a painful experience for any sentient creature. It lasts for about 10 minutes. Being subjected to a vacuum is painful, as is dismemberment by suction. . . . Again the time is about 10 minutes. Hypertonic saline solution causes what is described as "exquisite and severe pain" if, by accident, during an abortion, it enters subcutaneously the body of the woman having the abortion. It is inferable that the unborn would have an analogous experience lasting some two hours. . . . If a child survives pros-

taglandin poisoning, it will suffer impaired breathing and cardiac action. [In the fetus we may infer that] such impaired
functioning is ordinarily experienced as painful.[1]

Noonan argues that our society has advanced morally to the
point where we are unwilling to add suffering to the death sentence
in all situations except that of aborting the human fetus. We spare
dying animals from pain. Rapid and effective measures to end life
are used with cattle. The use of decompression chambers for dogs is
defined by law. "Can those who feel for the harpooned whale not be
touched by the situation of the salt soaked baby?"[2] Even in cases of
capital punishment we ask whether lethal injection is more merciful than the electric chair.

The ethic presented in these pages will agree with Noonan's
point and argue that, if abortion practice is to continue, new modes
of pain-free death by abortion must be discovered. It is possible that
we have widespread antipathy to the practice of abortion not so
much because we cherish life and seek to shield living beings from
pain but because we have deep guilt about our general disregard,
even destructive contempt, for the children of the world. Witness
the My Lai incident and the high infant-mortality rates in our own
cities. In adding the requirement of excruciating pain to abortion or
agonal labor to childbirth, we seek to assuage our own guilt. Otherwise, why are we such a right-to-life culture prebirth, yet callous
toward those same lives once they are born?

On the other hand, Noonan's position can be seen as an oblique
argument opposing the act of abortion per se. Indeed, throughout
his writing, the thoughtful Roman Catholic jurisprudentialist has
made that clear. Here we contend the moral question becomes more
complex. Surely there are situations where continuing a pregnancy
would produce more suffering than terminating it: the rape victim,
the eleven-year-old child, the mother in such fragile physical or
mental condition that the full course of pregnancy will profoundly
wound or kill her. Here the tough old Hebrew notion of the fetus as
potential aggressor (Rofer), armed to inflict harm, is valid, and we
are justified in countering this assault with defensive abortion in
the name of sparing a vulnerable one from suffering. Indeed, a rational calculus of suffering and redemption will lead us, as we shall
see later, to a policy where both the simplistic pro-life and pro-
choice doctrines are rejected in favor of an ethic that genuinely honors life and avoids suffering.

WRONGFUL LIFE/WRONGFUL BIRTH

A second line of reasoning on the abortion issue, one that also relates to our reflection in the last chapter about shielding the fetus from parental abuse, is the issue of "wrongful life" and "wrongful birth." The fundamental point of jurisprudence in these unprecedented cases is that one should not have to proceed through pregnancy without knowledge of knowable inherent risks and flaws. Morally speaking, the point is grounded in an ethical and an epistemological value. The ethical value is that prevention of suffering to the nascent life and to the family is good. The epistemic point concerns responsibility in the face of known and predictable outcomes. Do we have the right to give birth knowingly to a severely handicapped infant? Both arguments, it will be noted, devolve on the issue of suffering and the prevention of suffering.

The legal question is, Do children or their parents have a claim to recover damages against a physician or genetic counselor who fails to detect a genetic or hereditary disorder of malformation in time to abort the baby? The deepest jurisprudential, moral, and even metaphysical questions are whether there is such a thing as the injury of continued existence, or whether in any circumstance it is preferable "not to be" than "to be."

This new concern has emerged as science rapidly confers on us the ability to predict whether an infant will be born in an unhealthy condition, either sick at birth or prone to become sick later. The number of conditions that can be known through the glance into the fetal window and the accuracy of the prediction of morbidity (injury) increases every day. When techniques which include amniocentesis, ultrasonography, and chorionic villus biopsy are combined with laboratory analysis such as chromosome visualization and eventually gene delineation, an ever more accurate portrait can be drawn. Like the old polaroid pictures, which developed into focus before your eyes, we are now being presented with a vague but slowly defining picture of what a future life will be like.

An early case of wrongful life involved a mother who had contracted rubella during pregnancy (*Gleitman* v. *Cosgrove*, 1967). The baby was born with severe handicaps. The ruling and dissenting opinions reveal interesting ethical reflection focused on the themes of harm, suffering, and redemptive possibility. In deciding that the court could not award damages, it observed:

> In order to determine their [the parents] compensatory damages
> a court would have to evaluate the denial to them of the intan-
> gible, unmeasurable and complex human benefits of mother-
> hood and fatherhood and weigh these against the alleged
> emotional and money injuries. . . . When parents say their child
> should not have been born, they make it impossible for a court
> to measure their damages in being the mother and father of a
> defective child.[3]

Another perspective on suffering is expressed in Justice Jacob's
dissent. "While the law cannot remove the heartache or undo the
harm, it can afford some reasonable measure of compensation. . . .
Surely a judicial system, engaged daily in evaluating such matters
as pain and suffering . . . should be able to evaluate the harm which
proximately resulted from the breach of duty."[4] Subsequent cases involving Down's syndrome, hereditary hearing defects, and inherited
polycystic kidney disease have recognized legitimacy in the point
that parents should have been warned. The question of awards and
damages is still confused, since various states have enacted legislation declaring "wrongful life" appeals invalid.

The cultural value struggle that lies embedded in the "wrongful
birth" questions is more important than the "litigation fascination" it reflects. Shall we screen all beings that draw near to birth
into our world? Have we arrived at such clear and convincing ideas
of what constitutes "normalcy" or "affliction" that we know who
to turn back, who to detain, and who to allow to come on in? The
modern acceleration of abortion, resulting from the *Roe* v. *Wade* decision of 1973 in the United States and other laws around the world,
has exerted a massive denial at the threshold of life in this world.
The haunting question that remains is whether the alleviation of
suffering and the enhancement of life or the retreat into autistic life
is the central value.

A failure in our philosophy of suffering has led to this massive
confusion in ethics. Enlightenment philosophy since J. S. Mill has
counseled the avoidance of pain and the maximization of pleasure.
Today we have identified a range of pains that are unbearable or that
we feel we need not bear—pains mostly defined by technological
capacities to eradicate them, capacities which, at the same time,
cause other suffering. Since the prevalent philosophy has denied the
perennial philosophy of courageous fathoming, bearing, and sharing
of suffering and has counseled, instead, withdrawal and escape, we
have been left bereft of interpretive concepts and active disciplines

to confront suffering. We have responded by fashioning a chain of denials and escapes—pushing the human spirit into greater and greater impoverishment—culminating in a massive denial of death and the frantic worship of death-forestalling technology.

ABORTION AND THE ETHICS OF COHUMANITY

This life denial is most unconscionably expressed in the legalized and medicalized abortion practice of recent decades. Rather than calling to our attention this impoverishment of the soul and diminution of responsibility between persons and across generations, both religion and philosophy vacillated. Moral thought in this era concentrated on the language of rights, libertarian prerogatives, and feminism. All of these rationalizations depersonalized the human fetus.

Rights. The weary verbiage of the abortion debate most often used terms such as *right to decide, right to life, right to privacy, rights over one's own body,* and *fetal rights.* Actually it came somewhat as a surprise that a world that had largely abandoned the biblical, classical, and Enlightenment understandings of divinely endowed, natural, and inalienable right would resort to rights language when it sought to formulate philosophical wisdom for the age.

The language of rights was used by sides to justify a pseudorighteousness and to veil a deep sense of tragedy beneath. Those who used the term *right to life* glossed over the profound tragedy of a whole generation of young women which had been enticed by a promiscuous age, still found themselves without satisfactory contraception, were put upon by irresponsible men, and were abandoned either to illegal abortions or to the better hope, a more permissive legal and medical policy. Those who promoted the "right to choose" had to admit that we had severely eroded our respect for the most defenseless and vulnerable beings in our midst. Women especially knew this pathos because of the silent affinity their bodies had with such helpless unborn and because of the similarity of their plight. Both camps negated these counteremotions and forced the issue into the doctrinaire abstraction of cold and hard principles and away from the personal sadness that ensued with either course of action. Philosopher Daniel Callahan writes that, if we abondon respect and protection for the most vulnerable among us, "the most fundamental of all human rights—the right to life—will have been subverted at its core."[5]

Rights doctrine is the way human societies express their respect for persons. As Pope John Paul II said:

> America, your deepest identity and truest character as a nation is revealed in the position you take toward the human person. . . . The best traditions of your land presume respect for those who cannot defend themselves. If you want equal justice for all, and true freedom and lasting peace, then, America, defend life. The ultimate test of your greatness is the way you treat every human being, but especially the weakest and most defenseless ones . . . those as yet unborn.[6]

Rights language has a certain virtue and a certain danger. On the one hand, it holds before us the requirement of esteem and respect and places upon us the obligation not to harm. This respect and restraint is not contingent in one's reputation, on whims of affection or disaffection, on economic merit, or on influence. On the other hand, with the demise of a theological and philosophical basis for society, we are not secure in our doctrine of inalienability or inviolability of rights, and we therefore speak of rights being conferred instead of being guaranteed by commensurate responsibilities. This hesitation allows for the abrogation of rights when it entails hardship to provide them, and it encourages selective suspension of rights, especially to those whose voices cannot be heard.

Liberty. The central philosophical principle that has been asserted in the abortion debate is not a right but a liberty—the freedom of choice. Drawing on the spirit of the libertarian tradition of the English and French revolutions, the Lockean notion of civil government, and the modern advocacy movements of those who were formerly subjugated and exploited, a new accent on free choice was fashioned in a zone called the right to privacy. It is a freedom from and for: freedom from domination of the state by religion and oppression from any vested interest. It is also freedom for life, speech, movement, and work. The doctrine of freedom has also become ambivalent from a moral perspective. In one sense, freedom is the most fundamental of human rights. Without some range of liberty, life itself loses its value. In the end, another person can never be forced to do something against his or her will. One can refuse, lie down, stop eating, commit suicide. There is something of a bedrock finality to human freedom. The worst tyrannies have to find some way to seduce, satisfy, or sublimate the free will of a people. Freedom is also exhilarating. It is the delight of fully human existence, the essence of creativity and power, the noblest requirement of reason, a feature of the divine image that dignifies our life.

But freedom is also an empty value. Content needs to be poured into it. We should not be left free to kill or not to kill. Our freedom makes sense only in the context of meaningful values. Freedom is fulfilled more by generosity than gratification. The most ebullient freedom can be hellish slavery. Humble service can be perfect freedom. Liberty lapses into libertarianism or libertinism when it tears itself away from human goods and values. When freedom becomes defined by hedonist values, it quickly infringes on the freedom of others. Indeed, our whole modern society, enamored as it is with freedom, is basically constructed on dialectics of freedom and subjugation. My prosperity is fashioned on the impoverishment of others. Cheap goods require that, somewhere, someone offers cheap labor.

Since nascent life makes its abode within a woman's flesh and since some necessity (e.g. hyperfertility) intermingles with her free choice in the inception of life, in the early phase of impregnation she should be free in most cases to terminate the pregnancy. The sense of utmost seriousness should accompany each tragic choice. A sense of grief, lamentation, and general societal mourning is completely appropriate as loss and suffering is absorbed and vicariously healed. In general policy, in the first trimester our ethical system would concur with Callahan:

> Abortion should be legally available on request up to the 12th week of pregnancy. . . . Abortion is justifiable under a variety of circumstances [for our purposes these will be outlined later in the chapter]. . . . It should always be undertaken reluctantly and with a strong sense of tragedy; . . . The humane society could be one in which women are neither coerced to go through with pregnancies they do not want nor coerced by social, economic, or psychological circumstances into abortion. . . . I accord the right of women to control their procreation a high status, as a crucial ingredient of the sanctity or dignity of life.[7]

Rights and freedom doctrines, as part of the fabric of our society which accords great value to individuality and community, lead us to understand abortion as a serious challenge to both the sanctity and dignity of life. Resolution, the transformation of this tragedy into redemptive transfiguration, will require efforts from many directions, including:

developing safe and "believed in" contraceptives;

strengthening home, church, and school as sex and value educators;

developing social, economic, employment, and housing programs that hold out hope for poor young people;

strengthening adoption programs, especially of children born to poor and minority mothers;

removing stigma and offering honor and support to single women who keep their babies.

Such a constellation of efforts will be able to diminish gradually the call on abortion. They are appropriate programmatic responses to the philosophical themes of rights and freedom.

Feminism. Philosophy assumes two tasks in its contribution to social morality. In the analytic task it demands precise argument, careful distinctions, and justification of positions taken. Sorting out issues, showing the meaning of language, and pointing to inconsistencies in argument is an important function of moral philosophy. Philosophy has also rightfully assumed normative tasks and advocated just and good causes. One of the advocacy issues is feminism. The value contends that women's needs and rights have been denied and their interests suppressed. A special emphasis is needed to right past wrongs. In one sense, feminism may be a heresy. Heresy is defined as a truth exaggerated; masculinism is a heresy, as is communism, idealism, and materialism. They are all ideologies which take a valid idea and exaggerate it out of proportion. When the claim is made that abortion is the *exclusive* concern of a woman over her own body, the exaggeration of heresy and of false feminism is evident. Certainly, the baby, the father, and the woman's society is also involved.

PERSONHOOD

Exaggeration can be expressed by overstating or understating the reality. The ruminations of philosophy about the personhood of the fetus tend toward such understatement. Even an erudite treatment of the concept of person, such as that which we find in Michael Tooley,[8] still argues that personhood is an attribute, in complete disregard of the Western moral tradition of the Greek and Latin writers who developed the doctrine of persona. Engelhardt and Fletcher, in their impressive treatments of the concept of person, also argue that personhood is achieved by the acquisition of certain traits or qualities.[9] In their desire to advocate the feminist prerogative in the abortion debate, these philosophers, and indeed most writers in the analytic philosophical tradition, seek to diminish the claim of the fetus to fully human status. As Oliver O'Donovan has shown, this is to do violence to the Western tradition of the concept of person. "The concept of 'person' . . . in both its Latin and Greek form, was set in opposition to a qualitative analysis of what it is that gives us our identity."[10]

In the classics of Western literature such as Augustine of Hippo's *On the Soul's Beginnings,* the mystery of self-transcendence behind birth and beyond death is always held open. Though not unequivocally committed to doctrines of soul preexistence and immortality, anthropology that has come under the influence of Christology redefines human being and personhood in a radically new way. The passion of God for the human soul precedes and succeeds the concrete historic existence of each particular life, thereby bestowing ontic status, identity, and moral worth. This revolutionary concept of the person is reflected in the awesome passage "Before I formed you in the womb I knew you, and . . . appointed you a prophet" (Jer. 1:5 RSV).

The philosophical arguments supporting the availability of abortion, though possessing considerable merit, do not establish the case if we allow an ethic that reaches behind and beyond the imperatives found in natural human reason. The main philosophical directions of moral reasoning about abortion present a compelling case for moral justification of the practice. Review of these positions also document for our study the indispensable contributions of the philosophical perspective to a comprehensive ethical system.

The primary principles of philosophical ethics that bear on the abortion issue are autonomy, individuality, and happiness. Let us explicate these values with reference to some leading philosophical thinkers and then contrast them with countervalues that arise elsewhere in our ethical system: values of sacrifice, communality, and suffering. In this section, I will draw heavily on the insights of ethicists Lisa Cahill and Michael Tooley.[11]

A pervasive doctrine in modern philosophical ethics in general and in the abortion discussion in particular is *autonomy.* Taking the lead from Immanuel Kant and the European Enlightenment, the liberal tradition has positioned autonomy and noncoercion as the preeminent value. Tooley notes that liberal views on abortion which prevail in philosophical discourse mostly hinge on the view that an essential characteristic of being a person is self-determination. Since there is only one person involved as a primary party to an abortion decision, the mother's autonomy prevails.

If, however, as even Kant acknowledged, the central fact of morality is the interaction of an autonomous self with other selves and the gauging of the imperative by the good of the community of selves, then the essence of ethics is not self-affirmation but the adjudication, reciprocal compromising, and sacrificial accommodation of autonomous desires to the concerns of those others with whom one's life is bound up. Cahill argues that "respective rights must be defined in relation to one another. . . . Where those rights can conflict, neither can be absolute. The rights of both are limited, but still significant."[12]

Autonomy is a precious value. It needs to be vigorously taught and protected, especially in a world that tends toward homogeneity and absorption of the self into mass psychology and policy. In medicine, autonomy is also a crucial value, especially in situations of consent to experimental treatment and decisions at the end of life. The value cries out for the kindly balance of sacrifice in situations where other persons are integrally involved, situations like organ transplantation, receipt of scarce resources, and abortion.

A second accent of philosophical ethics related to autonomy is *individuality.* Although many schools of philosophy emphasize the one and the many (e.g. utilitarianism and Marxism), the emphasis of the analytic tradition in general is on individual reasoning and valuing and on the value of the personal rational being. No higher value exists in creation to which individual value should be subsumed. Alan Donagan draws on the teaching of Kant.

> The ground of the fundamental principle of morality [*oberstes praktischen Prinzip*], according to Kant, is that rational nature exists as an end in itself [*die vernünftige Natur existiert als Zweck selbst*]. From this ground it obviously follows that no rational being should ever be used merely as a means . . . but always as an end. . . . Every rational creature is to be respected as such . . . every human being is to be respected as being a rational creature.[13]

Here we see why the modern abortion crisis has forced us to depersonalize and even dehumanize the fetus and position primary active responsibility in the mother. But again, in the Enlightenment age, when the moral imperative was to cut loose from all tyranny over the self and when the spirit of the age was to reject all forms of incorporation of the self into some collective (ecclesial or economic), the fitting ethical response was to affirm individuality. Indeed, this emphasis must remain unshaken today. Modern conditions also require that we see individual good always bound up with communal value.

This enhancement of the doctrine of individuality is found in the complementary doctrines of corporeality and communality. Corporeal thought moves us beyond the dualist and Cartesian strains of anthropology, which have us think of the body as bad or inferior or radically separated from the soul, thereby reducing flesh to mechanism. The view which thinks of the fetus as an invader, a foreign tissue, or an appendage is not possible with a more corporeal view of the body. Cahill develops this point by quoting Janssens: "That we are corporeal means in the first place that our body forms a part of the integrated subject that we are; corporeal and spiritual, nonetheless a singular being. What concerns the human body, therefore, also affects the person himself."[14] This view, which enriches our understanding of human being by bringing historical, social, and biologic qualities to bear, also lays the foundation for seeing ourselves not only as singular beings but as part of a more communal body. We are always incorporated into the greater wholes of communities. We bear names which symbolize our link through generativity to the past and the future. We appear in families, and our life is always associated with a circle of others who nurture us through growth, accompany us through livelihood, and bear with us toward death. Ethics in some fundamental sense involves values that emerge from this matrix and not from sheer individuality.

A final theme of recent philosophy as it ponders abortion is actually an ancient motif that has close affinity with the moral system we espouse in this volume. The goal of life, philosophy contends, is pleasure, or *happiness*.

As the ancient and classical philosophers reflected on the beatitudes and vicissitudes of life, two truths came into focus. It became clear first that the primary ambition of the human organism was survival, protection, self-enhancement, achieving pleasure, avoiding pain, and establishing contentment and happiness. This was evidenced by observing brute human behavior and by studying tracings expressed in drawing, ritual, and narrative. Second, at the very moment when moral reflection engages the human mind, a reservation arises about this value of happiness. On the one hand, people observe that a life lived in pursuit of pleasure finds diminishing returns, since satisfactions create an endless cycle of greater needs for gratification. On the other hand, the moral soul—that conscientious part of us which ponders what *ought* to be—questions the worthiness and excellence of pleasure or happiness as a primary goal of life. Since life steals pleasure from us and since we ultimately yield life itself over to death, the thought crosses our mind that happiness must not be all that there is to life. A dialectic, therefore, emerges in the philosophical venture itself as some thinkers accent reveling in pleasure (hedonists, Epicureans), and others, conversely, accent renunciation (Stoics).

This tendency of philosophical principles to generate contrary emphases led Hegel to posit a fundamental dialectic of the human spirit and to propose that each of the dominant principles of ethics is understood most fully when we see it as part of a full-orbed complex, a rainbow with poles and an intermediate span of color variation. Justice as a phenomenon, for example, gravitates between the poles of vengeance and mercy. Autonomy moves through valences toward sacrifice. Reason tends to anchor concrete decisions on values poised between such radicals.

Today our pleasure-craving and pain-avoiding culture cannot come to rest even at this point of moral equipoise. We disavow failure and difficulty and shun sacrifice and burden sharing. If philosophy does have a predominant temper in our time, it is the utilitarian one of optimizing pleasure and avoiding pain. The cost-benefit and risk-benefit calculus is the value system that most persons, organizations, and institutions feel is the final truth about ethics. This presumption is usually rehearsed ad nauseam and not refuted by those who teach ethics in business, law, and medical schools. What passes for ethics in city halls, government task forces, college classrooms, and high-school bull sessions usually comes down to: "Does it work?" "What will I get out of it?" "What's the kickback?" "Will it leave me liable"?

Hard choices like abortion force us to look at the weakness of pleasure-obsessed ethics and see the salutary potentials found in suffering and solidarity. Callahan writes:

> Hard times require self-sacrifice and altruism—but there is nothing in an ethic of moral autonomy to sustain or nourish those values. Hard times necessitate a sense of community and the common good—but the putative virtues of autonomy are

primarily directed toward the cultivation of independent self-hood. . . . Hard times need a broad sense of duty toward others, especially those out of sight—but an ethic of autonomy stresses responsibility only for one's freely chosen, consenting-adult relationships. Whether suffering brings out the best or worst in people is an old question, and the historical evidence is mixed. Yet a people's capacity to endure suffering without turning on each other is closely linked to the way they have envisioned, and earlier embodied, their relationships to each other.[15]

THE PHILOSOPHICAL COMPONENT OF ETHICS

These accents of contemporary philosophy which bear on the issue of abortion—autonomy, individuality, and happiness—open for us the more general discussion of the philosophical component of human ethics and the rational faculty of the moral soul. At the outset we recognize that all ethics, from ecological to eschatological, are processed through the instrumentality of reason. We could, indeed, even speak of apocalyptic, theological, and eschatological reasoning (what have been called the revelatory modes of insight) as facets of moral reasoning. The capacity of the human mind in its cognitive, as opposed to connative, branch—the input of the higher sensorium, sight and hearing, intuition, inductive and deductive science, theoretical and practical reason, reflection upon cumulative experience, memory, common sense and prudence, wisdom in its experiential and intuitive sense—all these facets of the jewel of the mind contribute to the intellectual component of ethics, or moral reasoning.

The first function of philosophy is to activate the critical/analytic intellect. Values and beliefs need to be questioned, examined, and justified. In this sense, philosophical reason serves as a clearinghouse for values. It subverts and discards prejudicial, stereotypical, and to some extent, unworthy values, although one should not attribute normative discrimination to the critical intellect. Other beliefs and values it verifies and validates when it finds them coherent, plausible, and, to some extent, universal. Values are different from facts and are not established by conformity to some empirical criteria of verification. A belief or value can be justified when it is not refuted by any other channel of truth, when it is not completely idiosyncratic, when it claims some authority with many people, and when it commands loyalty and activates responsibility. Value judgments inhere in each of these criteria, of course, but in concert they form a body of evaluative mechanisms to assess the adequacy of any belief or value.

Earlier in this volume we argued that society should have a background and a foreground ethic. The deep ethic would ponder all the dimensions of ethics that we propose on our spectrum. The surface ethic in a pluralistic and secular society must of necessity concentrate on philosophical, legal, and other features of the middle range of perspectives. Here passion must withdraw as, in some sense, truth and compromise become the rule. In the public forum much more attention will be given to the process of ethical contention and resolution than will be given to ethical substance. At this point moral discourse such as that provided by philosophy and law, free from apologetic and passion, will serve us well.

The minimalist, procedurally focused ethic that can operate in a pluralistic society according to *consensus fidelium* and in an era of concern for "rights" and "duties" will attend to values such as autonomy, beneficence, nonmaleficence, fidelity, and justice—to use the well-worn pentad. Each of these values will be called on in its most customary and, therefore, most superficial sense. It will also be invoked mainly for its procedural import. The biomedical ethic that springs from the philosophical source is best described by Tristram Engelhardt.[16] Let us briefly sketch the character of these five philosophical values as they are transformed by the companion components of our system.

To return once again to *autonomy* in our scheme, self-interest will be defined as it interplays with all of the components of value. My freedom is enhanced by environmental protection and ecological equilibrium. Attuned to apocalyptic dynamics, I discover self-fulfillment participating in nature's agonal spasms toward fulfillment. Self-determination is found both in responding to the biologic "wisdom of the body" (Cannon) and in transcending its brutish impulses. True freedom is to live animated by the finer affections among the many (love and hope) and by the nobler mutation of each of the emotions (agape instead of lust, hope instead of despair). Autonomy is protected by both law and society and is tempered by the public interest. The historical element of ethics links freedom to the conditionedness of the past and the openness of the future. The example of history also gives normative shape to freedom. Selfhood is both grounded in religious faith and relinquished in devotion and final reunion with God. In eschatology the ultimate possibilities of freedom are glimpsed, possibilities presaged under the conditions of existence.

Beneficence and *nonmaleficence* can be similarly explored. In the system we are sketching, these ethical principles go close to what Richard Alter considers in "What Is the Substratum?" What is the nature of the altruism and "other concern" that rises from the rational mind? A certain "in-group" altruism and even a naturalistic peace (*The Peaceable Kingdom*) is found among the animals and in the biologic dimension of human morality. Disinterested agapic self-giving sacrifice is inspired by the divine spirit. But what nature of care and beneficence, and what manner of restraint of maleficence, rises from the rational mind itself? At one level, calculated enlightened self-interest prompts consideration for others, and avoidance of retaliation gives rise to "nonharmful" behavior. Immanuel Kant anchored benevolence in the rational soul as practical reason perceived the categorical imperative. This rendition of the ancient and universal Golden Rule found that we respect and kindly treat others not out of pure self-interest (although that element is present) nor out of selfless good will (that element is also present) but rather out of a necessity of reason. We are to treat others benevolently and refrain from harming others so that each action is capable of being universalized.

The exploration of morality on which we have embarked would find another source of kindness in natural reason. When we look upon another person in pain or suffering, we are moved to help, unless our mind is contorted by apathy or morbid glee at misfortune. In other words, one of the natural functions of the mind is identification and empathy. Though the thought does not consciously form but remains in the unconscious, part of the response is asking, "What would happen if I were the one who needed help?" Of course the desire for self-adulation or the desire to be seen performing a good deed is also present. More probably, aid in distress is a natural and necessary response of the knowing soul to the crises and sufferings of life we all share.

The relevance of this insight of philosophical ethics to the abortion question is somewhat troubling. From a fetus the claim "I want to live" or "it hurts" cannot be heard or known. Suffering in the fetus cannot be presented directly to our cognitive awareness except perhaps by some act of mental reconstruction or imagination. While analytic reason cannot prompt one to benevolent disposition, various normative commitments within a philosophical system can commit a person to this doctrine.

In this light it is not surprising that moralists who focus on the philosophical channel of insight should, in the case of abortion, not heed any claim from the hidden life but respond to the voice that can be heard and the need that can be known—those of the mother. Philosophical treatises which do affirm some "fetal value" because life or personhood is present "in potential" usually are not convincing. The ethics of natural reason respond best to the cognitive channels of awareness. Reason, as Hume showed, is empirical, and even innate mental structures, if Kant is correct, need to be activated by experience and transcendence.

The point of appeal to the senses (seeing and knowing) as a precondition of moral response also casts light on another issue in abortion. Some critics have argued, somewhat in the spirit of surrogacy, that women who wish to abort should just carry on awhile, deliver the child, and then hand it over to adoptive parents who have been preselected and are anxious and ready to have the child. Would this not solve two great problems—abortion and the shortage of babies for adoption? The proposal forgets that, once a mother holds the baby and looks in its eyes, she can never let it go. The bond of seeing and holding fashions the morality of knowing. In one famous case a mother gave birth to a child and then gave it up for adoption because she could not afford to care for it. Six years later the court gave her permission to pick up the body of her child, whose adoptive parents had abused and killed her. The courts returned custody and the privilege of this last embrace to the natural mother. The case vividly shows the impossibility of the idea that children are interchangeable.

Beneficence and nonmaleficence are values which are known and not foreign to reason, but they rely on recognition and are thus somewhat fragile. More powerful grounding for the virtues of care are in biology itself, especially the genetics of temperament and disposition; in psychology, especially the ethical yield of nurture and training; and in theology, where gifts of the spirit, including compassion, are bestowed even over against nature, nurture, and rational intent.

The same is true for fidelity. It is surprising and gratifying to see on recent lists faithfulness and trustworthiness added to the principles of philosophical ethics. (See, for example, the work of Andrew Jameton and the nursing ethics film *Code Gray*). Again, Kant anchors moral habits like truth telling and promise keeping within moral reason. But is it reasonable never to lie and always to keep one's promises? Why does it make sense? Kant might argue that lying and breaking promises fractures a cosmic moral order and lays bare future transactions to moral chaos. He might say that fidelity fulfills inner propensities of our selves as moral beings. One always wonders whether Kant is appealing not to reason alone but also to the religious pietism of his Lutheran worldview, where divine mystery—the will of God in the soul, even eschatological elements (damnation or salvation)—provides stimulus for fidelity.

In our system fidelity is a cardinal virtue. Grounded in all of the enticements to ethics, being there and staying there, even when one is tempted to abandonment or promise breaking, is the fully moral response to an unpredictable and terror-filled world. The ethic we propose also transforms the virtue of justice into a somewhat richer principle than is customarily found in philosophical treatments.

CONCLUSIONS ON ABORTION

Philosophy is the love of wisdom. Philosophical ethics, in its deepest sense, is a passion of the mind wherein the noblest insights of reason and logic, as well as gratuity and caring impulse, are affirmed. Philosophy displays a certain disposition about the world. Justice as a principle of ethics contains within its own conceptual boundary this rich breadth of meaning. As we bring this particular parameter of ethics to bear on the question of abortion, we quickly see the respective virtues of formal ethics, impassioned ethics, as well as the broader comprehensive system we have proposed.

If one follows the formal categories and logic of philosophical ethics, one usually concludes that abortion is acceptable, especially if the principium employed in that system contends that in freedom all is permissible that cannot justifiably be proscribed. Engelhardt, for example, holds that "one harms no person either by not conceiving that entity or by aborting the body from which it would develop."[17] Other ethics will emphasize condolence, conceived not only as empathy with the burdened woman but with the fetal human being whose life is threatened. A philosophical ethic tempered by justice and mercy will arrive at a nuanced ethic of abortion. A ship that must always sail in troubled waters will seek to avoid the treacherous shoals both of a "right to life" and a "right to choose" ethic. In conclusion, we submit a moral view more subtle but therein more responsive to pain-bearing responsibility.

ABORTION: A MORAL POLICY

This ethical analysis requires that we differentiate abortion cases along a moral spectrum. It is simplistic to say that abortion is always right or always wrong. Even though philosophy demands consistency and the law requires uniformity, more subtle decisional criteria should be applied when our choices involve human beings. Therefore, we need to distinguish among differing situations and admit that there are times when the technique of abortion must be used. In the public policy arena we need to develop an ethic of reason and prudence. Then in a nuanced way we can assign value or disvalue to a given case according to some balance of the principles to beneficence, nonmaleficence, justice, and freedom.

A suggestive grouping of cases might be these: abortion would be *strongly advised* in incest, child rape, and cases where profound genetic defects (e.g. Tay-Sachs, Lesch-Nayan syndrome) are present or the pregnancy or delivery is life threatening. Abortion is *permissible but not obligatory* in coercive out-of-wedlock pregnancy, situations where pregnancy offers a physical or mental risk to the mother, moderately severe genetic or congenital abnormalities discovered in the fetus (e.g. Siamese twins, spina bifida, Down's syndrome). Abortion is *permissible but discouraged* in illegitimate pregnancies, mild and treatable genetic or congenital accidents (e.g. harelip, cleft palate). Abortion is *proscribed* for reasons of convenience, population control, and sex selection. Who should be the judge to say whether any of these conditions exist? The answer is obvious. The final choice should lie with the mother and father, together with medical and pastoral counsel. The law should convey general contours, but abortion should not be seen as a criminal act unless the specific case falls under this last category.

This proposal suggests that neither "right to life" nor "freedom of choice" doctrines satisfy. Both abandon the subtleties of freedom and conscience. Our society appears to be groping for some nuanced abortion policy that will more appropriately honor our cultural values of "sanctity of life," "freedom," and "justice." We must reject the morally simplistic reduction of this complex of issues into the "right to life" and "life begins at conception" configuration, on the one hand, and the equally absurd "freedom of choice" doctrine, on the other. We need some carefully nuanced public policy which avoids the dangers of being restrictive or conducive for the tragic interim until completely reliable and trustworthy modes of contraception are available and used. In this tragic interlude our sense of judgment and our schemes of ethics will be severely put to the test.

6 Epistemic Ethics of Knowledge and Ignorance:

GENETIC HEALTH

Schafe können sicher weiden, wo ein guter Hirte wacht.
J. S. Bach, Cantata No. 9 (Sheep may safely graze)

The good shepherd counts his sheep. If one is missing, he returns to the grazing lands or mountain crags to rescue it. Counting is an act of judgment, occurring in that zone of mind that cognitive scientists call computational neuropsychology. Carrying a lamb (*amnion, agnus*), one way to speak of being a mother, is also an act of pastoral judgment. Today the mother with child, her husband, and the specialists who attend her are confronted with awesome computational and pastoral responsibilities. Genetic probabilities must be weighed. Amniotic probes such as amniocentesis, ultrasonography, and chorionic villae sampling yield to the moral

93

psyche—to the calculating, judging faculty of our soul—some certainties, some probabilities, some possibilities, and some impossibilities. This body of knowledge and speculation now provides a data base for decisions. We always must act with the benefit of knowledge and the bane of ignorance.

The fact that we live *Anno Domini* does not make our judgments easier. If anything, decisions become more perplexing because we living A.D. have been robbed of that moral innocence which the pagans enjoyed. Abortion and infanticide became problems for us in ways they were not for the Greeks and Romans because we have been given a new comprehension of suffering and redemption. Assimilating the life-honoring moral power of Mosaic Judaism and the pathetic sensibility of exilic Judaism, a new ethos has been fashioned. The era inaugurated by the appearance of Jesus Christ into world history and the people inspired by the Christ spirit now look at life and death, pain and birth, and being with child in a new way. Though this residue of value is severely threatened and hardly negligible in our time, it still has moral impact.

To develop further our discussion of the ethics of natality, we must look at the capacity for moral calculation framed within the context of knowledge and ignorance. This mode of judgment we will call epistemic ethics. By "epistemic" ethics we mean the calibration and calculation of risks and dangers rather than Plato's contrast of *epistēmē* (factual knowledge) and *doxa* (opinion).

THE MORAL SIGNIFICANCE
OF KNOWLEDGE ABOUT LIFE

In the garden of paradise stand two trees—the tree of life and the tree of knowledge of good and evil. In our time these trees have been grafted into each other. We are now beginning the long, arduous, and morally problematic quest for detailed knowledge of the human genome, the master blueprint for life itself. Like the paradise garden trees, this quest is not one of pure intellectual intrigue, it is a search for power. What we seek is ameliorative knowledge— knowledge to improve, to rescue, to help. It is knowledge that is now being pursued with urgency. Not only is there commercial and economic competition and a frantic race among nations, there is an urgent desire to gain an upper hand at diagnosing and treating the devastating diseases that continue to wreck havoc on the human species.

When we speak of ameliorative ambition, we are talking about *gnōsis* (knowledge) in all of its forms. We desire preventive gnosis. How can two parents who are carriers for sickle-cell anemia assure that their child will not have the full-blown disease? We desire precise diagnosis. How can we see into the germinal, cellular, and chromosomal basis of life? How can we see through the extents, the lineaments, and the cross-references of genetic conditions? We desire prognosis. Where will this lead? How will it become manifest? What, if anything, can be done about it? The human genetic project is a moral response to the crisis of suffering affecting humankind. It embodies the desire to redeem this tragedy.

Armed with a new group of tools and techniques, it has now become possible to begin the mapping of the entire human genetic repository, amounting to some 100,000 genes and 3 billion units. This means locating and defining the composition of each gene within each chromosome. The epistemic and ameliorative package that is opened will be mixed to be sure: "Some of the uncovered genes will be of inestimable clinical value (perhaps allowing us to prevent or cure disease). Most will have unknown functions. . . . Others will raise as many problems as they seem to solve."[1]

The main tool which opens this door to knowledge is known as a DNA probe. These single strands of radioactively labeled or chemically tagged DNA have known sequences of nucleotides which interlock with their precise counterparts. A DNA probe of nineteen or more such bases will almost certainly code for a unique segment of DNA, a gene. Whether the entire map will be plotted or whether genes having medical importance will be given priority is a decision yet to be made. If the genetic material that renders one susceptible to Alzheimer's disease is on the twenty-first chromosome, the same one which anchors the Down's syndrome anomaly, we may start our probes on these more pathological foci. On the other hand, we may decide to undertake an undiscriminating look at the whole bed of inheritance, sending out sensors for benign as well as malign traits. We may search out all provocateurs, even those which influence size, eye color, intelligence, and disposition.

For the time being, we seem to be concentrating not on those genes which predispose to late-onset chronic disorders (e.g. Alzheimer's, cancer, hyperlipid anemia) but on those carrying early morbidity which are amenable to prenatal diagnosis. These disorders include cystic fibrosis, polycystic kidney disease, Down's syndrome, sickle-cell anemia, thalassemia, hemophilia B, and Duchenne's muscular dystrophy.

Initially, it appears likely that we will gain knowledge about the genetic basis of human disease. This will be beneficial, but only partially so, since the genetic foundation of diseases constitutes one of four of the elements in the etiology. For diseases actually to take hold and achieve their morbid and mortal effect, there usually also has to be (1) *interaction* with other genetic and biologic processes; (2) *penetration* through to an actual manifestation of disease (e.g. someone may have a mild penetration of a syndrome, an arbitrary grouping of signs, called ectodermal dysplasia, which in some persons is life threatening, with major system compromise, but in a given case may present itself only as missing teeth, fragile mucous membranes, thin hair, and fair skin); and (3) *stimulation* of some external or environmental insult or stressor (e.g. toxin, virus, or experiential trauma) which issues in the onset of the disease.

Some diseases seem to have obvious and uncomplicated genetic bases—the single-gene disorders, for example. These will most likely be the first group to be understood and resolved in some manner, either by reduction of incidence through genetic counseling, by selective abortion, or by some corrective mode of therapy. Hemophilia B, for example, can be dealt with in three ways. The affected fetus can be found in prenatal diagnosis and be aborted. The fetus or child can be identified and clotting factor VIII can be introduced. This will not change the genotype but will offset the symptoms (bleeding) in the phenotype. Third, a genetic therapy such as gene replacement may someday substitute a good gene for the faulty one.

Another group of diseases and disorders do not set themselves up so nicely on the genetic display and will involve a multifactoral genetic basis and therefore a more involved resolution. Cancer, heart disease, and various forms of mental disorder (e.g. schizophrenia) will fall within this group. Not only will the genetic ground of these disorders be more difficult to locate precisely, but the ancillary triggers (penetrance, insult, etc.) will be more complicated and elusive to control. A moral difficulty that will present itself with this range of diseases and disease proclivities is that elimination will be easy (abortion), phenotypic protection will be complicated and perhaps be of uncertain efficacy, and genetic transformation will be very difficult and cost inefficient. Eradication will be easier and cheaper than edification. We will very likely choose the easy route.

Finally, a fund of genetic knowledge is available about who we are and what we are becoming that even defies designation as disease or disorder. Human conditions such as immunologic vigor, intelligence, personality, and the code for aging will very likely present themselves to our scrutiny and then force the question, Now what are we going to do?

Two observations come to mind as we view this decisional horizon. First, it becomes clear that quantification, calculation, and mathematical cognition as modes of decision analysis will become more crucial to ethics. Brute facts are the groundwork, the givens of ethics. The placing of a category of epistemic ethics within our spectrum of consideration indicates the importance we attach to this vector. Mathematical and utilitarian intelligence alone, however, will not suffice for ethical judgment. The modality will need the enhancement of all of the other norms on our continuum.

What of the moral import of these amniotic probes? As we begin to use them, we find we have launched our Niña, Pinta, and Santa Maria—our ships of life, life giving, and life protection—into new and uncharted waters. Where we will land, in paradise or hell, is not known. We have asked a question, begun a probe, sought an answer, which, like the sampling of fruit in the paradise garden, will leave us never thereafter the same. Though the arrogance of the enterprise is troubling, the more troubling aspect of this new power is the occasion it presents for irresponsibility. Alasdair McIntyre asks with his bitter but powerful wit whether, at the conclusion of this egomaniacal and comfort-seeking endeavor to design our descendants, we might find the good sense to design a person who, unlike us, had no desire to design his descendents.[2]

Leon Kass remarks poignantly:

> I was conceived after antibiotics yet before amniocentesis, late enough to have benefited from medicine's ability to prevent and control fatal infectious diseases, yet early enough to have escaped from medicine's ability to prevent me from living to suffer from my genetic diseases. To be sure, my genetic vices are, as far as I know them, rather modest, taken individually—myopia, asthma and other allergies, bilateral forefoot adduction, bowleggedness, loquaciousness, and pessimism, plus some four to eight as yet undiagnosed recessive lethal genes in the heterozygous condition—but taken together, if diagnosable prenatally, I might never have made it.[3]

Knowledge enhances our capacity for goodness, for apathy, and for maleficence. Moral outcomes will be determined by our funda-

mental inclinations. Heightened knowledge and power have not provoked enlarged measures of courage and caring within us so much
as they have fostered the desire for easy solutions, quick fixes, and a
general retreat from challenge. All these diversions from paths of
responsibility and these abdications of duty have become possible
because of a defective worldview, resulting in a faulty sense of
moral destiny. We have come to construe the human task on earth
as one of alleviating hassle and burden rather than seizing upon the
bequest of knowledge and power as a chance to heal a sick world,
repair a broken human family, and fashion a kingdom of justice and
righteousness. Let me be concrete. Why do we choose to use the
therapeutic powers of genetic science and DNA recombination to
create a human growth hormone so that people, embarrassed by
their shortness (as people are by baldness and wrinkles, age and ug-
liness), can become taller? Why do we not rather use this power to
create vaccines for malaria, Chargas, or schistosomiasis, diseases
that aggravate millions of the earth's peoples into constant sickness
and early death?

There is something very questionable about the eugenic project
when we submit it to moral analysis. In moral reminiscence, we
need to relearn the lessons of Nazi, Russian, and early American
eugenics. We need to cleanse its unworthy fascinations and emphasize the salutary directions, all in the light of more carefully defined
prohibitions and goals discovered in a moral vision more splendid
and compelling.

GENETIC THERAPY

The moral vision of which we speak is animated by pictures of a
peaceable kingdom which indeed relates to our scientific knowledge
and technological skill. The new world we seek is not some spiritu-
alized inner-induced escape or Castanedic bliss; it is a world of concrete undertakings which aid human helplessness, debility, brevity,
and harshness of life. Jesus the healer, whom our civilization calls
the Annointed One, came bringing sight to the blind, ambulation to
the lame, sanity to the deranged, and release to the oppressed, all in
the wake and spirit of a moral regeneration, a new power of redemptive existence.

A halting step in the biologic ramifications of this redemptive
direction is found in the therapeutic possibilities of genetics. Three
manifestations of a new peace on the horizon are genetic medicines,

fetal therapy, and gene therapy itself. Regrettably the embryonic en-
trée of genetic medicines is sullied by commercial exploitation and
unclear indication of need. Since science and technology can advance only in the areas that are ready for progress, we need to examine morally not only each new development but the overall goals
of the project.

In the American free-enterprise system, substances of medical
therapy are produced in terms of maximum salability and mini-
mum liability. The first therapeutic substance produced by gene-
splicing was therefore, not surprisingly, a vaccine to prevent swine
from getting dehydrated from persistent gastroenteritis. The American motto Bring Home the Bacon, we may assume, is the reason
that pigs get the first shot while again millions of humans worldwide continue to suffer the devastations of malnourishment and
dehydration, including mental retardation from similar chronic
infestations.

Most of the vaccines will likely be mass-produced one day by
DNA recombination, creating the virtue of a more general availability and widespread distribution than is available now with the cum-
bersome and expensive extraction techniques. Insulin and interferon
are among the widely mentioned substances for early exploitation.
We may hope that a range of antiviral vaccines, including swine en-
cephalitis vaccine for countries like China and HIV vaccine for the
AIDS-infested West, will become available. In addition to this, a
wide range of hormones can be genetically manufactured, including
somatostatin, somatotropin (a growth hormone), interlukin (a cancer cure?), calcitonin, relaxin, cortisone, gastrin, and thymosin,
which plays a role in orchestrating the immune response. Add to
this the other body proteins—such as the neuropeptides, which give
rise to many euphoric and dysphoric mental states, and body
proteins in the blood like clotting factor VIII and serum albumin—
and a rather promising future begins to take shape. We may be
able to mix human genes with sheep and grow these hormones in
the serum of the innocently grazing creature. Most of the crucial
processes of life are triggered and mediated by protein-induced cellular processes, all of which will eventually be better understood
and replicated.

An intriguing development of natal therapy in the light of our
discussion of abortion is the inception of the new art of fetal medicine. Though these initial acts are not in the field of sophisticated
genetic therapies but rather are basic manipulations (e.g. detoxifying
fetal kidneys, draining a hydrocephalus, transfusion-exchanging a

blood supply), they presage a vast array of measures to correct injuries, perhaps even offset deleterious genetic or congenital injuries, before a baby is born. The moral irony comes into focus. If the fetus is now a patient, observed and attended with such immaculate care, can the practice of abortion long continue? The cruel sequence of cases where babies are aborted alive and sent into intensive-care units for management and treatment reflects the horror of our moral ambivalence on this point.

Part of our moral quandary that we are confused about is our ameliorative and redemptive obligation. As noted in chapter 5, we are not sure whether our task is to alleviate suffering by doing away with the source of pain or by transforming that challenge into a new opportunity. What we do in the case of the "flawed" fetus or the aborted fetus illustrates this bewildered moral eschatology. On the one hand, we heroically intervene in utero to save the life of the fetus and correct serious disorders. Fetal medicine promises to become a lively horizon of therapy. We seek to redeem a troubling situation. On the other hand, we sometimes experiment on or crassly use a fetus, supposedly "bringing some good" out of a no-win position.

In one clinical case a woman had conceived a baby from her husband, who was dying of kidney failure. She informed her physician that they wanted to use the baby's kidneys to save the father's life. Would the doctor and the hospital perform the procedure? As an added cruel twist, she said if they refused, she would abort the baby anyway. "Then what good will come?" Often we seek to extract redeeming value out of tragedy. The psychodynamics of organ donation in brain injury cases often focus on the desire of those who remain—say, the relatives of the auto crash victim—to find some purpose in the tragic circumstance. More and more today, parents—for example, those who give birth to anencephalic babies—demand that some good come out of this tragedy. The now on, now off decision to use the diagnosed anencephalic newborns to donate hearts to babies with congenital hypoplastic left heart syndrome exemplifies this.

In a similar case, a medical ethicist was asked an equally bizarre yet agonizing question. The woman asked whether she could be artificially inseminated with sperm from her father, who has Alzheimer's disease. Her plan was to abort the fetus and transplant its brain tissue into her father's brain. She had heard of the early experimental data on fetal-cell transplants and the value of adrenal cell implants for Parkinson's disease. Dr. Robert Gale, of Chernobyl bone-marrow transplant fame, argued, "All of us that work in fetal research feel that, if someone decided to have an abortion and gives permission, it is all right to use that tissue to help someone else."[4]

Two views come into play in this discussion of exploiting the use of aborted fetuses for tissue donation and other experimentation. Both hinge on an interpretation of some wrong done or some tragedy experienced and the possibility of bringing from that untoward event some redeeming value. The first view, espoused by fetal scientists, decries the act of abortion, tongue in cheek, and says, "If this sad thing has to happen, let's get some good out of it." Those opposed to such fetal research and exploitation contend that a grievous wrong has been done in the abortion and add, "Let's not compound it by doing more harm." The latter view is also tinged with a spirit of retribution which does not allow that any good effect assuage the guilt of the abortion.

Both of these views err in the sense that they remove the issue of evil and suffering from the human beings who are involved and render it an abstract issue. Pain should be gauged in terms of real harm to actual human beings, those alive or yet to be born. The concrete powers of calculating danger, harm, and injury afforded by empirical and epistemic evaluation will help us to sharpen the question of harm and take the issue away from those who would exploit tragedy or foster further suffering by intensifying guilt.

The larger issues of genetic therapy and the broader concept of genetic improvement will be explored in chapter 7, on eugenics. Our purpose in this chapter is to examine the specific question of genetic diagnosis of fetal cells, especially those sloughed off in the amniotic fluid for diagnosis, and the attendant question of ameliorative action. We have mentioned how information becomes known and also some things that can be done in light of the data. We have considered postmortem utilization of aborted fetuses in conjunction with fetal therapy, only to point out the varied moral meanings of redemption applied to such phenomena. Genetic knowledge and the derivative therapeutic quest is driven by impulses of avoidance, amelioration, and ambition, all of which reflect underlying metaphysical and metaethical commitments. John Fletcher puts the matter in perspective. He speaks pastorally to persons who are going through the perplexing crises of knowledge and ignorance, satisfaction and guilt, doubt and faith.

> I believe that the pain and suffering that you experienced was not lost in the rivers of time. Your suffering makes a difference to God, who not only gives unfailing courage to face the unknown, but who also creates the limits of our freedom to learn

in such a way that more good than evil can eventually prevail. If a child is ever cured of a genetic disorder by a gene therapy that is the result of scientific research, the event will not have removed the evil that was done to you and your family. But you and I will have understood more about the goodness of God and the meaning of participation in God's emancipating work. God's abiding intent is emancipation and not punishment.[5]

What we can know and do is a judgment *in amnion*, a judgment or confrontation which evokes profound background meanings and immediate pragmatics.

EPISTEMIC ETHICS

There are two principal ways that the calculating and computational powers of the human mind enter into the ethical equation. Calculation of the risk-benefit ratio of a given decision or action has been an integral part of ethics from the beginning of time in virtually every moral system. Though the distinction between what are counted harms and goods are themselves value laden, it is generally agreed that some measuring of results comes close to being a value-free concomitant for every moral decision. This is not to argue that mathematics defines morality. Joseph Fletcher writes, "Call it what you will—mathematical morality, ethical arithmetic, moral calculus—we are obliged in conscience to think of benefits relative to costs."[6] Although we cannot go as far as Fletcher seems to argue in his "ethometrics," we can agree with him on the necessity of moral computation.

Second, the moral soul of individual persons and the collective will of a society always deliberate and calibrate on the basis of knowns and unknowns. A certain moral advance is achieved when we set aside arbitrary and subjective feelings and wills on a given issue and submit them to an objective standard on which all can agree, a baseline quantitative standard of measureable elements. Let us develop the ethics of such knowledge, ethics in an epistemic mode, with reference to the questions of genetic analysis of potential offspring.

In one sense all ethics is a matter of weighing and measuring. When Burton introduced precise scales into the corn market of Oxford in the seventeenth century, he ushered in a new era of justice. Economics, which we will discuss in more detail in chapter 8, as political ethics, involves the acts of sharing, distributing, equalizing, and allocating within a house, a coinhabited place. When we ask whether a response or reaction is fair, be it a human action or even divine justice, we draw on the ancient meaning of marketplace, or fair. Is that which is meted ("metered") out fitting in terms of what has been presented?

The whole notion of epistemic ethics is based at least in part on a Newtonian notion of causality. It assumes that every action has an equal and opposite reaction. If the cue ball traveling at a certain speed and direction hits the eight ball on a leveled pool table, the reactive movement of the eight ball is predictable. In genetic counseling, parents are told that if this sperm carrying this chromosomal package with this dominant genetic disease fertilizes this ovum with a genetic package also dominant for that disease, this will occur in the offspring. How do we know? Two reasons: scientific deduction and historical precedents. $A + B$ always equals C, either because of some inherent capacity of A and B to combine to form C or because, when observed many times, it always happens. "If you do that you know what will happen." This is the moral injunction that arises from this assumption of logic and experience.

The most helpful version of epistemic ethics is found in the new discipline of clinical reasoning, or decision theory. This insight into ethical judgment, developed at the juncture of the two disciplines psychology and philosophy, helps to clarify both prescriptive theory (how decisions should be made) and normative theory (what should be decided).

One of the leaders in the field, Arthur Elstein, argues that decision theory has taken on new relevance in medicine because of its ability to bring two elements to bear on clinical judgments, elements hard to integrate into decisions but indispensable to clinical wisdom: value and uncertainty. These dimensions are crucial, first, because clinician judgments, the determinations of doctors and nurses, for example, are value laden, often in conflict, and not, as we would like to think, always objective and scientific. In a similar fashion the patient brings a rich array of values and belief to the encounter in the clinic. As Foucault has shown, the empirical concentration of the clinic is somewhat in conflict with the value concerns of therapists and patients.

Values, at least quantifiable values like morbidity (injury in its measurable aspects) and mortality, can be factored into decision trees. Probability theory can also be added in to assess the efficacy of alternate procedures. An example of such epistemic analysis is described by Elstein. "The issue is what protocol would be most efficacious in the treatment of head injury. Three strategies are offered: (1) Operate on everyone to avoid missing any intracranial bleeds. (2) Do a neurological evaluation, then CT Scan only those with positive signs. (3) Do skull films on all patients; scan patients with positive films and operate on patients with positive scans; go to strategy (2) for those with negative scans."[7] If mortality alone is used as a sole criterion, the application of Baye's theorem, 2 ×2 tables, and decision trees will tell you which strategy will be best, that is, which will minimize the incidence of death and misdiagnosis. The example makes clear the strengths and limitations of statistical, mathematical, logical—indeed, all epistemic—approaches to ethics. Where a good can be measured and an undesirable outcome quantified and when the data that has been gathered clearly secures benefits and avoids harm for significant proportions of any cohort, then such clinical decision analysis is of obvious value. When crucial factors are not measurable or are only partially measurable and when collective data do injustice to individual members of the group, the process does not suffice and must be supplemented by other avenues of ethical insight.

The ethical genius of decision analysis is also its drawback. The specificity of this approach, achieved by limiting the factors under consideration and ruling out many other variables, gives an answer in hard numbers. If theorems, formulas, and equations can embrace a significant enough range of pertinent data, very helpful conclusions may be reached. But ethical decisions seldom lend themselves to such close delineation. Wider and wider concentric circles of influence impinge on the volatile center. Many factors which are known cannot be measured. Many relevant factors cannot be known. The desire to control variables may be a disguised version of an attempt to control ambiguity, which is to deny the richness and depth of moral situation and ethical responsibility.

Let us take a concrete example of genetic decision making to illustrate the virtue of epistemic ethics. A woman who is thirty-nine-years old and becomes pregnant can receive a fairly specific percentage figure of her risk of having a Down's syndrome baby. If the factors of socioeconomic status, race, husband's age and health, number of pregnancies, and the like are weighed, a figure—say, 5 percent chance—can be arrived at. Wanting more certainty, she can wait until ten weeks of gestation and have an amniocentesis. Now the chromosome analysis can tell conclusively one thing—whether the trisomy 21 condition is present. But the problem remains—how deep is the penetrance? Are injuries to major organs present? Is intelligence severally affected, or will this person be capable of a regular education? We do not know whether the mother is capable of deciding on and following through with an abortion. Similarly, could this family tolerate the presence of an affected child? In addition to these limitations, the full ethical question—Is this right or wrong?—is not answered, only the utility question, Is it workable?

Thus it is not surprising that, just as our ability at mathematically based clinical judgment has reached a zenith, we also witnessed a widespread discussion of medical fallibility.[8] Increasing knowledge ironically brings with it the awareness of how much we do not know. As significant as the knowledge and power side of epistemic insight is for ethics, it is no more important than the side of ignorance and impotence. In the ethical system we are proposing, virtue or moral strength is based at points on competence and control and at other points on receptivity and humility. Let us examine the moral impact of fallibility.

FALLIBILITY AND MORALITY

In a very searching and illuminating volume, Charles Bosk, a sociologist, reports on his eighteen-month field study at Pacific Hospital as a participant-observer on the surgical service. He initially observes that "medical decision making is a probabilistic enterprise." Yet even though the enterprise is based on the assumption that we know x (disease) and therefore do y (intervention), "only rarely is it the case in which the physician can say 'this patient has x and we must do y.' "[9] Whatever may be the nature and depth of his or her uncertainty, the physician is usually forced by the patient's condition to act before that uncertainty is resolved. In most cases the doctor must proceed to do something with greater or lesser uncertainty.

Bosk continues to explore the fascinating social context and configuration of action that medicine has fashioned for itself with considerable direction by society. Indeed, though the ideal determinant of medical decisions would be epistemic and technological certainty, the actuality of profound and pervasive fallibility and ambiguity has instead fashioned a milieu of "reasonable" action undergirded by dispositions of remembrance, understanding, and forgiveness. Here we see the epistemic voice of ethics calling back to its precursor of prudential wisdom (philosophical) and calling forward to its successors—remembrance (historical), forgiveness (theological), and hope (eschatological).

In genetic decisions the force of guilt, shame, and retaliation (e.g. wrongful-life suits) that is let loose when the pretension of knowledge fails is enormous. After unnecessarily aborting the living child of a patient who deeply wanted the baby, Dr. David Hilfiker, in an unusually candid article in the *New England Journal of Medicine,* says he was unable to confess the misdiagnosis and mistake and that "even months later, . . . I never shared with them [the parents] the agony that I underwent trying to deal with the reality of the events. I never did ask for their forgiveness. I felt somehow that they had enough sorrow without having to bear my burden as well."[10] Only the amplification of an operative ethic behind and beyond the strictly utilitarian can serve us well so as to redeem rather than condemn the participants in such hard choices.

The moral underlining of epistemic ethics, decision theory, and talking with patients about diagnostic and prognostic probabilities is not so much certainty and fallibility as it is honesty. We all feel the need to convey certainty, even in the face of gnawing doubt. This shrinking back from hard honesty usually is an attempt to avoid or alleviate pain in the other or in oneself. Jay Katz has addressed this problem in one of the important recent books of clinical ethics, *The Silent World of Doctor and Patient.* He has just been talking with a surgeon-colleague about the variable judgments of contemporary medicine on the best treatment for breast cancer. As with so many medical conditions today, there exist several acceptable treatments, each with a certain array of statistics (often conflicting), risks, and benefits. The surgeon rationally and mathematically reviews the options in discussion with Katz. But with his patient something completely different transpired.

> At the beginning of their encounter the doctor had briefly mentioned a number of available treatment alternatives [to his patient]. He added that he had done so without indicating that any of the alternatives to radical surgery deserved serious consideration. Instead, he had quickly impressed on his patient the need for submitting to his operation. I [Katz] commented that he had given short shrift to other treatment approaches even though a few minutes earlier he had agreed with me that we still are so ignorant about which treatment is best. He seemed startled by my comment but responded with little hesitation that ours had been a theoretical discussion, of little relevance to practice. . . .

> He then asked me what I might have done instead. I told him
> that I would have first clearly acknowledged our ignorance
> about which treatment is best . . . and proceeded to lay out in
> considerable detail all treatment modalities . . . (offering my rec-
> ommendation only after she had indicated her inclination). . . .
> He responded that . . . most of his patients would not tolerate
> such explorations . . . such conversations would cause them
> anxiety and considerable pain. . . . I was particularly struck by
> his real concern about not causing his patient any pain. Yet I
> also silently wondered whether he would have been equally, if
> not more, pained by having to converse with her about his cer-
> tainties and uncertainties as to the choice of treatment.[11]

Again we see the crucial role that the ambition to alleviate or
ameliorate pain has in our ethical judgments. We seek to avoid the
difficult confrontations of honesty and sharing because we cannot
believe in the redemptive possibilities of the human soul under the
divine spirit. In contradiction to the full heritage of our moral traditions, we feel that the burden of sharing will be exhausting and
not exhilarating. To care, share, and bear one another's burdens is,
in the modern mechanical-electrical imagery, to "burn out." In reality, deep wisdom knows that such compassion "lights my fire."

Standing in the rich ethical heritage which is ours, fallibility
can be acknowledged as a liberating source of humility and interdependence and therefore of moral power. We are not commissioned to
know and fix all, but rather to care attentively. This, of course,
means rigorous use of the predictive and conclusive side of our
moral psyche. But fundamentally it means concession to the ultimate wisdom of a higher order. When Herman Muller sounds his
apocalyptic alarm on genetics, pleading with us to exert strong
knowledge and power over "load" accumulation in the gene pool,
Paul Ramsey cautions: "Anyone who intends the world as a Christian or as a Jew knows along his pulses that he is not bound *to
succeed* in preventing genetic deterioration, any more than he
would be bound to retard entropy, or prevent planets from colliding
with this earth or the sun from cooling. He is not under the necessity of *ensuring* that those who come after us will be like us, any
more than he is bound to *ensure* that there *will be those like us to*
come after us."[12]

We are not obliged to perfect life and the world but only to do
right with what we are given. Epistemic ethics constitutes an essential building block in the foundation of our ethical structure. Its

weight helps hold the moral edifices erect. Yet, like the other building blocks, it depends for its integrity on the companion blocks to
either side. Let us conclude this chapter by appropriating epistemic
ethics and its companion moralities to some specific questions of
genetic health.

THE ETHICS OF GENETIC HEALTH AND DISEASE

In 3.5 percent of the cases where prenatal diagnosis is sought,
bad news is received (the rest receive good news). In this relatively
small percentage of cases, the diagnosis of some problem is "positive." Down's syndrome, for example, is found in the fetus. Now
abortion must be considered. This abortion is morally problematic
for two reasons. On the one hand, there might seem to be great justification for abortion because something is wrong. This assumption is carried to the point that some genetics centers will insist on
seeing evidence that there is a willingness to proceed to abortion
before fetal diagnosis is offered. If some evidence of ambivalence is
found in the parents, the center might propose that the family come
to some willingness to abort before the test is performed. In our
litigious age clinics do not want parents to regret a decision later
and sue.

The other side of the "selective abortion" problem is its obvious discrimination. If the doctrine of causality has any bearing on
human decisions, it might be considered discriminatory to end a
life because of some flaw or defect. John Fletcher admits that it
might be argued that "the use of prenatal diagnosis tends to set
apart certain fetuses as deserving of abortion and thus treats fetuses
unequally and unjustly."[13]

Epistemic ethics would argue in this case that a new factor has
come into play. Once we take in hand the probe of knowledge, like
the forbidden fruit of the garden tree, we are now responsible for
what we have come to know. No longer innocent, we now knowingly give birth to a defective child. Putting aside all of the ridiculous notions of the child's some day bringing suit against the
parents for giving it birth, we do have a serious new dimension of
responsibility once we demand that the face appear on the amniotic
mirror. The larger ethic, however, will contend that such knowledge
is not harsh in its requirement but rather a gentle encouragement to
us to do what seems proper to honor life, avoid harm, and, as lies
within us, effect redemption. Some families may decide they cannot
bear the responsibility of birthing a severely deformed child. Others

may seek more definitive tests to assess the actual extent of the anomalies. Other families may decide they can bear the outcomes and proceed to birth. In all instances moral counsel and support should be extended to the couple without retribution or penalty.

Another area where genetic knowledge joined to clinical technique takes shape in public policy and affects the fate of persons is that of discerning disease susceptibility. Some hundreds of diseases or conditions are already known to have biologic markers. With these markers, it is argued, we can look into the future and see the specific maladies that persons will succumb to. If the discovery is found in utero, appropriate measures may be taken. The screens or probes more likely will be used on adults. Prospective employees may be tested for their susceptibility to developing certain forms of cancer—whether they have, for example, the pulmonary cellular characteristics to develop lung cancer if exposed to smoke or other noxious insults. DNA probes will one day designate those who are at risk for recurrent infections, periodontal disease, arthritis, back ailments, and AIDS.

It appears we are being drawn irresistibly toward a day when minute fragments of inconclusive knowledge shrouded in vast clouds of ignorance will come within our view. We will be called on to make decisions about persons' health, their productivity, their potential, their future. Will we strengthen the battery of safeguards, protections, and options of appeal for people, or will we use the occasion of this newfound knowledge to clean house, reduce costs, minimize risks, and further diminish the fragile liberties so recently and sacrificially gained?

The proper end of genetic medicine is the detection and treatment of inherited disease. To eradicate the bearers of present flaws or biologic markers embarks us upon a new voyage not unlike the classic eugenic voyage to which we will next turn. The desire to cleanse the pool, like the desire to eliminate suffering or eradicate death, is simply the ameliorative ambition become vicious. As Hannah Arendt has written, natality ethics is the opting for hard love and helpful work, a grounding of our moral (indeed, human) existence in order to save, heal, and redeem persons, not to escape into painless and effortless bliss. "The miracle that saves the world, the realm of human affairs, from its normal, 'natural' ruin is ultimately the fact of natality, in which the faculty of action is ontologically rooted. It is, in other words, the birth of new persons and the new beginning, the action they are capable of by virtue of being born. Only the full experience of this capacity can bestow on human affairs faith and hope."[14]

7 Historical Ethics of Eugenics:

STERILITY AND SURROGACY

Memory, turn your face to the moonlight
Let your memory lead you
Open up, enter in
If you find there the meaning of what happiness is
Then a new life will begin.

A. Lloyd-Weber, "Cats" (after T. S. Eliot)

No other people has ever shown so strong a compulsion to explore their origins.
The Bible gives constant examples of the probing historical spirit: why, for instance, was there a heap of stones at Gilgal? This passion for aetiology, the
quest for explanations, broadened into a more general habit of seeing the
present and future in terms of the past. The Jews wanted to know about themselves and their destiny.

Paul Johnson, *A History of the Jews*

We now see where we get our fascination with generativity, genetics, eugenics, and destiny. The convictions of the children
of Israel underlie Western science and ethics. A pervasive historical dimension, a sense of time and movement, of nature and destiny, has entered our intellect and conscience and has indelibly
shaped our moral soul. We continue to explore the range of natality
questions, especially our efforts to make babies as we want them,
overcoming constitutional impediments and managing with quantitative and qualitative values the fertilization, gestation, and presentation of new lives. This chapter will review a spectrum of issues

from an ethics conceived historically and then gathered within the larger system we are proposing. We will then consider the three remaining dimensions of moral reflection—sociological, theological, and eschatological. Through the functions of remembrance, faith, and hope, we now add elements which will enrich and mature our personal and collective conscience.

We have been exploring concerns where our generative and procreative nature has been perceived to be out of our control. In issues of being together and being with child, we asked whether human integrity could be maintained in the face of sexual power and the bonds established by that power. In the population explosion too many children were being born. In AIDS, abortion, amniocentesis, and handicapped newborns, the sexual-procreative process somehow raged uncontrolled, and we had to deal with some tragic aftermath. Our discussion now deals not with ignorance and impotence but with increasing power and control over the presentation of new life. Part of this increased control is the ability to overcome "natural" impediments such as infertility or sterility. We now suppose that these new technological abilities are tokens of a new authority over age-old inevitabilities. It is appropriate, therefore, that we now bring historical perspectives of ethics to illumine these newfound powers. From history we become aware of the conditional and determined character of our actions. History also speaks of our ability to transcend the past by virtue of coming to understand it.

The word *eugenics* is used guardedly. Scientists and therapists today eschew the term because of its pejorative associations and its painful reminder of the Nazi era. On the one hand, we now hold more modest ambitions about improving "genetic health" than did the eugenicists of the early part of this century. We know how complex the interactions are between human gene action, environment, and therapeutic interventions. Most scientists agree that it is foolish and presumptuous to set down rules for human breeding such as those which flourished forty years ago.

At the same time it must be recognized that modern biomedicine, like all creative human endeavor, stresses sheer power and originality as opposed to restraint, formalism, or conformism. Like the New York School of Abstract Impressionists, scientists today are artists. Pollack, Klein, Rothko, and Rosenberg sought unhindered expression. So do the sculptors of birth.

While it is uncertain whether or not we have in mind some grand eugenic project and ambition, it is certain that we do not share the sense of impending calamity and urgency that shaped the negative eugenics of an earlier generation. While few would deny that emphasis has shifted from positive to negative efforts, the alarmist words of Julian Huxley in 1963 would today find little support.

> The population explosion is making us ask . . . What are people for? Whatever the answer . . . it is clear that the general quality of the world's population is not very high, is beginning to deteriorate, and should and could be improved. It is deteriorating, thanks to genetic defectives who would otherwise have died being kept alive, and thanks to the crop of new mutations due to fallout. In modern man, the direction of genetic evolution has started to change its sign from positive to negative, from advance to retreat: we must manage to put it back on its age-old course of positive improvement.[1]

Huxley calls us to reassert an ancient and, he would argue, time-honored project of positive eugenics. Eugenic history and its driving ethic as this has been in resonance and dissonance with the traditional ethic of Western culture must first be examined in order to establish or refute Huxley's point. The questions of different modalities of conception and gestation and the new issues of fertilization, surrogacy, and innovative gestation represent new eugenic questions, for these make parents of those who are, in the state of nature, biologically unable to be parents. If we are to evaluate not our success in transcending nature but our wisdom in tampering with her laws, we must turn to those events which suggest "normative value"—how we should and should not live. Our technical powers do not decrease; so much greater then is our need to examine present and future by the light of our historical memory. Let us look at one example of intervention in the classic tradition of negative eugenics—the newborn PKU screen. This example will acquaint us with the elements of the question of which we need to be aware.

PKU AND THE NEWBORN SCREEN

In the disease phenylketonuria, a single gene disorder creates the absence of a crucial enzyme, allowing the building of a toxic load in the newborn and causing severe mental retardation. If the disorder can be detected by the newborn screen of the Guthrie test, the diet can be modified for phenylalanine during early life and the child spared from this loss. In New York City between 1966 and 1974, fifty-one PKU infants were discovered. Though screening all newborns during that period cost $1 million, even on a purely cost-saving basis the program was worthwhile. The moral obligation to uncover the disorder and modify diet was overwhelming, once the power to know and to do something became available. The compelling case for intervention and policy requiring screening became complicated only when the female children whose diet had been corrected started to arrive at childbearing age themselves. If they decided to have a natural child, they faced two problems. If they modified their own diet just before and during pregnancy, the child they carried might be normal, and then again it might not. The evidence is not in on that question. Should such women be forced by law or policy to be sterilized or to assume the difficult diet? On the other hand, the woman who was treated as a baby for PKU might opt to adopt or to have a baby by some other modality of fertilization and gestation, or she might remain childless.[2]

We see in the light of this case the new situation of eugenics. We can manipulate the child's life for the child's benefit or we can change something about the mother. Eugenesis—good beginnings—can entail either or both approaches.

EUGENICS: OLD AND NEW

Persons desire to "make babies" differently for one of three reasons: they cannot have children by the good old ways because of infertility or some other problem in the potential father or mother; they wish to improve on what is possible by some eugenic effort; or they do not wish the hardship of conception and or gestation and choose some alternative method such as surrogate pregnancy. The old eugenics were different in that they displayed a basic celebration of conception and a desire to do well through the generative process. Only recently, with the development of new technique, has the spirit of dissatisfaction and desire for radical transformation set in.

Our culture's belief that life giving must be done well finds its roots in Hebrew faith. Since divine purposes and human obligations have to do with the life and destiny, the birth and death, of persons, the kingdom of God or kingdom of heaven imagery in Hebrew Scripture translates into a eugenic and euthanasic picture.

I create Jerusalem to be a delight
   and her people a joy;
I will take delight in Jerusalem and rejoice in my people;
   weeping and cries for help
   shall never again be heard in her.
There no child shall ever again die an infant,
   no old man fail to live out his life;
   every boy shall live his hundred years before he dies,
whoever falls short of a hundred shall be despised.
....

My people shall live the long life of a tree,
and my chosen shall enjoy the fruit of their labour.
They shall not toil in vain or raise children for misfortune.
   For they are the offspring of the blessed of the Lord
   and their issue after them.

(Isa. 65:18–23 NEB)

Hebrew eugenics is rooted in the expectation of an age when infant mortality will cease and babies will be born whole and well. Hebraic hope means that we should draw heaven near and approximate in our world here and now that world where "no child shall . . . die an infant" and parents shall not "raise children for misfortune." We do this by generating new life with responsibility and care, by conceiving new beings as if we were cooperating with the divine Creator, and by seeing conception as a divine blessing. We must also care for the gestation of this new life with respect, for it is a life miraculously our own yet mystically not our own. We must provide dietary, hygienic, and psychological care both for ourselves and for that new, totally dependent person. We also create the social, economic, and political conditions for the eugenesis—the wholesome and healthy development of these new lives that have been entrusted to our community.

Our Hebraic heritage also shapes the pathos ethic, which is the reverse side of the ambition for wellness and perfection. Here, in the history of the Jews, we derive the sense which we make of suffering, which is the heart of the moral question of what evil we resist, what evil we abide, and how we find meaning in resignation. From the lamentation ethic of the Exile to the messianic ethos of the suffering servant, to the Holocaust literature and the meaning which the event has assumed in contemporary thought and value, Hebrew history provides a check to overweening eugenic disposition. We are to seek to be well, to honor the body, to exult in sexual power and procreativity—to transmit life whole and healthy and to live with gusto and gratitude all of our days. This praise of life which we offer in the Noachic covenant affirms that the story will go on until the Messiah redeems the creation and consummates history. But yet we acknowledge suffering, we understand that brokenness is often our lot, and we find redemption even in the midst of dysphoria, dysgenesis, even Holocaust. Job asks, "Why do the righteous suffer?" and Rabbi Kushner asks, "Why do bad things happen to good people?" Each question portrays an outrage, an uncanny undergirding hope that things should and will be different. The demand for justice expresses trust in the faithfulness of the One who brings all to pass.

Another root of our eugenic ambitions and dysgenic antipathies is found in classical civilization. Plato and the Greeks also had a eugenic ethic, frequently characterized as harsh and infanticidal. Indeed, it was morally debasing until it was transformed under apocalyptic Judaism and the impact of the Christian gospel. Yet, in Greece there was a fundamental humanism that desired procreative well-being.

Plato frames his ideal state as the golden mean between the warrior discipline of the militant Greek city-state and the pleasure-oriented Corinthian life-style. In *The Republic* the state regulates marriage, procreation, and childrearing. Plato's eugenic policy can be divided into three phases. First, there is an emphasis on securing maximal excellence in offspring by mating strong and intelligent individuals. This is done by planning and programming the meetings, friendships, and patterns of association of young adults. The "inferior" offspring of the guardians of the upper class are degraded and made to relate with the more modestly endowed offspring of the lower classes. At the same time, the gifted children of the warriors are given access to upper-class society. Wives of "like nature" are selected for guardians and legislators. The commonwealth includes communal housing and dining, and "the best of either sex" is to be "united with the best . . . as often as possible." Rulers determine the number of weddings, so that both the appropriate quantity and quality of new lives are conceived in order to sustain and invigorate the community.

Second, ideal matings are encouraged so as to bring forth children ("such fathers ought to have as many as soon as possible"). There is an obligation to transmit what we now know to be the genetic endowments of intelligence and competence to children so that the community will be strengthened and edified.

Finally, the last checkpoint for eugenic excellence is abortion and infanticide. Embryos of incestuous and other dysgenic conceptions are to be destroyed. Although the harshness of the Spartan policy of sex selecting is not found in Plato, we do sense a chauvinism that disvalues the lives of female children. Feminine infanticide was widely practiced. We can also believe that, had it been possible to identify them, Plato would have favored the destruction of sick and deformed fetuses, because the neonatal policy moves in this direction. While officers of the city take the offspring of "good parents" and raise them in the fold, the offspring of the inferior (and even of the better, when they chance to be deformed) are "put away in some mysterious unknown place as they should be."[3]

Modern ideas about eugenics began to take shape in the Renaissance, where utopias devoted much attention to the arrangements of mating, marriage, procreation, and childrearing. Thomas More, for example, saw public good as much more crucial to a commonwealth than personal wishes. For this reason children, although raised in the nurture of extended families (parents and grandparents), were the heritage and responsibility of the larger community. In a family that had too many children, for example, newborns were removed to another family. Like chicks that follow and feed from the mother first known, children were adoptable. Before a man and woman married, they were invited to view each other nude to screen for blemishes that would offend the partner or be passed on to offspring. In general, both the English and French utopias of the sixteenth and seventeenth centuries sought to find a balance between programmatic eugenics and spontaneity.

Utopian communities of the eighteenth and nineteenth centuries such as the Shakers actually implemented programs of sexual behavior and childbearing. It is no accident that these benign political eugenic utopias are followed by the horrific dystopias of the modern world. It was while visiting an Austrian monastery that Adolf Hitler formulated his eugenic programs very much in keeping with the racist and cultural-superiority mythology of nineteenth-century anthropology. Lysenko and the Russian eugenicists proposed programs for breeding a superior race. Herman Muller of the United States visited Russia and, with Julian Huxley, proposed programs to ensure that superior germ cells were united to assure in the coming society the presence of strong, compassionate, intelligent, and gifted individuals. Among other mechanisms, Muller and Huxley suggested that a woman bear one child by her husband, then be allowed to choose another sperm donor of her choice; this, it was thought, would facilitate the basic biologic and ethological impulse found among all animals whereby both the male and female exert some eugenic selectivity. The modern sperm banks where the depositors are medical students or Nobel laureates are vestiges of these early twentieth-century eugenic utopias.

The critical observer will see that all of the plans to build a more perfect race through positive eugenics are based on a diagnosis—or fear—that the gene pool is being polluted. Whether it be the adulteration by inferior stock, the contamination of racial and ethnic differences, or, in the case of Muller, the diseasing effect of deleterious genes (e.g. diabetes), the eugenicist believes that frightful deterioration of the human race is imminent if his or her programs are not swiftly enacted. Even today the IQ geneticists argue that inferior intelligence capacity is being transmitted much more rapidly than is genius, since the poor and uneducated have more children than do the new intelligentsia.

A severe condemnation and refinement of our historic eugenics emerges in the Nazi era. In 1933 Hitler's cabinet promulgated a eugenic sterilization law based on American examples. But this compulsory law went far beyond the laws of Virginia and California which the Germans emulated. Now all persons who suffered inherited diseases including "feeblemindedness," schizophrenia, epilepsy, blindness, drug or alcohol addiction, and a range of physical deformities were forced to be sterilized. The Reich's minister of the interior said, "We want to prevent . . . poisoning the entire bloodstream of the race." All this was thought to issue from the highest ethical motivation. "We go beyond neighborly love; we extend it to future generations. Therein lies the high ethical value and justification of the law."[4]

Beginning in 1934, physicians were required to report all "unfit" persons to one of the "hereditary Health Courts." By 1983 one-quarter of a million people, mostly designated "feebleminded," had been sterilized. Positive eugenic measures were also introduced to improve the hereditary stock, all the while the negative eugenics of this act of cleansing was going on. Subsidies were given to "strong" families which bore a third and fourth child. The economic and "Volkish" value of such procreation was stressed. In this spirit the somewhat comical Lebensborn movement was founded, where not the Jewish intellectuals and artists but SS officers were encouraged to father many children by preferred women, who were then offered special prenatal care in spalike homes.

The irony of the Lebensborn movement was, in fact, its dysgenic effect. Throughout the nineteenth and early twentieth centuries, it was assumed that German Jewry were part of the Aryan

race, an essential part of fashioning and improving the German national stock. It was only when extreme envy, fueled by a sense of
inferiority, shaped the anti-Semitism of "ill-bred" Nazis that the eugenic policies added "racial" characteristics to the sicknesses it
sought to excise from the body. In the Nuremberg laws of 1935,
marriages between "Jews" and "Germans" were forbidden. As Lifton and others have vividly pointed out, the eugenics and natal
policies of the Nazi movement in the early 1930s became the euthanasia policies of 1939. Now Jews were included in the class of the
physically and mentally disabled who were designated for death.

We have contended throughout this book that the drama of redemption and counterdrama of damnation form a metaphysical
backdrop for the manifestation of human good or evil. Noting the
connection of the German eugenic movement with the American
will help us see the universal tendencies to be disavowed. In 1936,
the year of Jesse Owens's Olympics, the University of Heidelberg
voted an honorary doctorate of medicine to Harry Laughlin, a sterilization enthusiast who directed the Eugenics Record Office at
Cold Spring Harbor, Long Island. When Laughlin received the honor
at the German consulate in Manhattan, he acknowledged the
"common understanding of German and American scientists of the
nature of eugenics."[5] What was wrong with this era which sought to
bring into being children of strength, beauty, and intelligence by
manipulating the processes of mating, conception, and selection of
special mothers?

In the first place, as Alasdair McIntyre has shown, the person
least to be trusted with the power of "designing their descendants"
are those so ignorant as to believe they can.[6] Quite often eugenics
proposals reflect the wishful longings of a disenfranchised and em-
bittered group who have been deprived of their inherent dignity or
otherwise stripped of the natural gratitude that every person and
group should have for their own existence. American blacks offered
little resistance to the sterilization laws of the 1930s or the Tuskee-
gee syphilis studies of the next decade. It was only in the 1950s and
1960s, when the civil rights movement and Martin Luther King activated a renewed sense of dignity and gratitude, that cries of genocide could be raised against the sickle-cell screening programs.

A second reflection that arises from this recollection of the old
eugenics was the unfortunate pairing of mental and physical conditions. While it is true that the most tragic expressions of dysgenesis
are those persons who come into our world with damaged or diminished powers of brain and mind, it is also the case that such persons

are least able to understand or object to what is being done to them—say, in the case of sterilization. When we begin to extend the categories of physical normalcy to the brain and mind and its qualities (such as intelligence, personality, disposition, and aggressiveness or passivity), we cannot defend our actions. The human mind, personality, or soul is a realm of profound depth and infinite variation. To claim that we know what is a healthy personality or normal intelligence or who is a worthy soul is to assert unimaginable arrogance and unacceptable discrimination.

A final critique that becomes clear as we view in retrospect the old eugenics was the ease to which it could be put to the service of political, racial, and even economic bigotry. Most communities of people which have any sense of cohesiveness practice some sort of eugenics, such as the matchmaking of twentieth-century Russian Jewish ghettos or planned marriages in Chinese villages. These efforts may be understood as natural law or biologic wisdom. Where these natural proclivities are joined to powerful technology and state jurisdiction, the danger arises that eugenics policies which reflect the rudest and most debased human impulses may predominate.

Both positive and negative values can be gleaned from the Hebraic and Hellenic roots of eugenic ethics as these are seen in the mirror of such a tragically tarnished history. An unmistakable eugenic mandate affirms that we are to do well in bringing children into the world, giving them as strong a birthright as is possible—a body that can thrive, a mind capable of delight, a spirit free to care and be creative. One of the purposes of human existence is to fulfill physical, mental, and spiritual potentials and, through moral commitments, to leave the world better than one found it.

We are also constrained so that in our freedom we do not knowingly hurt another or concur or conspire with other forces that would harm. Here the growing scientific capcities of knowledge and power convey an important eugenic responsibility. When we know something dangerous or deleterious can be transmitted to another, whether AIDS or a severe genetic defect, we surely have a duty not to pass it on. This responsibility will, of necessity, be graduated. Responsibility weighs more heavily not to conceive one who will be severely damaged, if that can be avoided, than it does to abort one that has been innocently conceived. One has more responsibility to help the severely injured newborn than to save an anomalous fetus that will miscarry or require an abortion. Gradations of knowledge and ignorance and gradations of severity appear along a moral spectrum. The 50 percent chance that a male child will be born with severe combined immunologic deficiency presents different responsibility than the remote possibility that the child conceived will develop cancer when he is sixty years old. The conception and delivery of a hemophilic child whose life can be spared with factor VIII (before AIDS, that is) or the birth of a child with hereditary hypercholesterolemia who could be managed with lovastatin is of a different moral order than delivery of a Tay-Sachs infant who will die excruciating death in the first years of life. There is an appropriate eugenic imperative to do as well as can be done in natality and not knowingly to harm. There is also the moral imperative to blend spontaneity and trust into our generative life and not place with grave seriousness the demand to be perfect upon ourselves or others. The scandal of moral self-righteousness demanding infallibility and the law perpetually scanning for liability can only leave us with a residue of undue guilt, compulsiveness, and sadness.

A final theme of value that can be derived from our moral heritage is the appreciation of not only spontaneity but diversity. The danger of all eugenic proposals is that they drive toward homogeneity. It is a short step from the desire to eliminate defect in the interest of normality to the desire to eliminate diversity in the interest of some norm. Anyone with scientific appreciation knows the value of hybrid vigor and the rigor of diversity, but technology and law thrive on regularity and uniformity. Indeed, any bureaucratic society seems to crave regularity for its own purposes of organization and administration.

Moral crisis thus ensues when value is placed on certain qualities and disvalue on other. Genocide is the moral evil of the quest to eliminate some ethnic or racial variation, but gene variation too is threatened. Various strains of feticide and infanticide are being pondered as we seek to identify and eliminate groups of children with certain syndromes, such as hemophilia. By careful lineage tracing and genetic counseling, one cohort of this species can be eliminated. By amniocentesis and selective abortion, we may in the near future initiate another assault. While at present a newborn cutoff is neither practiced nor contemplated, a cruel irony threatens in the short run nearly to exterminate the entire hemophiliac community. Because of contaminated clotting factor a few years back, some 90 percent of all hemophiliacs in the United States now are seropositive for AIDS.

In light of our moral motif of suffering, death, and transfiguration, the desire for pervasive normalcy reflects the desire for apathy, silence, stillness, disengagement, and (ultimately) nonbeing. Unwillingness to accept that which is different is part of the desire to reject that which drives us out of ourselves, that which illustrates the new (the word *monster* comes from the verb *monere*, to warn).

THE NEW EUGENICS: STERILITY AND SURROGACY

Now that fertility and fecundity have been reduced to a function, we find ways to revise, repair, and even replace that function. Leon Kass reminds us of the historical process by which we have come to see sexuality as a technology, infertility a problem to be fixed, and surrogacy a gestational option.

> Ancient Israel, impressed with the phenomenon of transmission of life from father to son, used a word we translate as "begetting" or "siring." The Greeks, impressed with the springing forth of new life in the cyclical processes of generation and decay, called it genesis, from a root meaning "to come into being." [It was the Greek translators who gave this name to the first book of the Hebrew Bible.] The premodern Christian English-speaking world, impressed with the world as given by a Creator, used the term "pro-creation." We, impressed with the machine and the gross national product (our own work of creation), employ a metaphor of the factory, "re-production." And Aldous Huxley has provided "decantation" for that technology-worshipping Brave New World of tomorrow.[7]

Fertility was once construed to be a blessing, even a divine visitation, and childlessness represented the status quo. Now infertility is a curse, and fertility a capacity to be regulated by human modulation. Yet, not only infertility but hypo- and hyperfertility are functions of population ecology, as the fruit-fly environment demonstrates. But should biologic necessity or theological gratuity constrain our decisions or behavior today? The yearning to have a child is intense. In the modern world, where options of finding or making a child are numerous, the desire to have one's own biologic child becomes strong, and couples seek to enhance fertility, stimulate or elevate subnormal fertility, or circumvent impediments such as fallopian-tube blockage.

To evaluate ethically this aspect of human experience, we need to assess both the desire to accept or resist the state of infertility and childlessness and the techniques than can be utilized to try to overcome the impediments. On the first question we certainly must find virtue in the act of accepting with magnanimity this limitation of life. We must also extol the courage and care exemplified when childless couples adopt a child, especially a minority or a handicapped child. The unwillingness to accept the limitation and the restless desire to find some way to have one's own child is morally neutral. The wish for a child may grow out of a generous heart, a healthy commitment, and a willingness to observe that joyful sacrifice of parenting which allows life's story to pass on to another generation. One can also imagine numerous unworthy motives that might be present.

Moral discrimination must be deployed as we evaluate the measures which are used to achieve birth along with the side effects and outcomes of those measures. The literature of ethics quite rightly concentrates on the specific measures of overcoming infertility: artificial insemination via donor or via husband, in-vitro fertilization, various measures of stimulated ovulation and spermatogenesis, surrogacy, and the frontier of cloning and extrauterine gestation. Before we offer ethical reflection on these specific measures, we need to recall the high dignity that history and our moral traditions have bestowed on the received grace of procreation. In most old and classic traditions of ethics, we find the accent of the biblical tradition which extols the privilege and mandate of having children. By bearing children the woman fulfilled her true purpose in life. The barren woman was looked upon with pity and even disdain (Gen. 16:4). The man was given the vocation—indeed, the mandate—to "raise up offspring," which were like arrows in a quiver or the glorious new shoots of an olive tree (Pss. 127:5; 128:3). By having children, we complete our being. To be joined to another in love and to have that love yield fruit is to draw forth a mystery that was meant to be. This is not to say that singleness and barrenness are a disgrace. It is a different vocation with its own particular purpose. But this new mania of liberal society—bachelordom and the singles scene—does not diminish in any way the crucial existential, social, and spiritual necessity of persons' becoming parents.

AID (Artificial Insemination Donor) and AIH (Artificial Insemination Husband) present no particular moral problems except to separate love from procreation, which not only severs a natural and normative conjunction but threatens the assurance of continued care. Where one of the conceiving parties is involved only by an anonymous donation, substitution must be made to complement the other parent in supply of care and nurture. IVF (in-vitro fertilization) has provoked a fairly large literature pondering the ethical issues. The issue of fertilized embryos which are then discarded has been raised. The issue of required parentage has asked whether single parents, gay or lesbian couples, or special groups might conceive and raise children. A major question at this point is whether the technique will be placed in the domain of private, for-profit business or whether it will be regulated in some way, under the care of university medical centers. A third series of questions has been raised with reference to experimentation, informed consent, and taking risks with the future lives of human beings who, by definition, cannot consent. Both Leon Kass and Paul Ramsey have raised the difficult question of defects that come into the nascent life.[8] Ramsey claimed that we should have permanently refrained from using this birth technology because the only way we could assure that such an enterprise would not harm would be to undertake unconscionable experiments on the unborn.

The moral consideration hones down to the crucial question of whether a joy and good to be achieved can justify dangers and wrongs afflicted. The temporal question arises, Can a potential good justify the possibility of a present violation? Are there intrusions into the very nature of life and life giving that can never be justified? A tremendous risk exists that we will avoid these deeper questions and allow "baby making" to become not Huxley's horror but a glib commercial technology. Such an apathetic retreat, an opting for detachment with an escape from both pain and responsibility, will bring not the hell of some final denouement but rather enduring dull sadness. The law of love and sacrificial care always finds itself in tension with the desire for ease and exploitation.

Perhaps the most poignant expression of this conflict of values is found in the practice of surrogacy. On one side stands the National Coalition against Surrogacy, led by Mary Beth Whitehead and aided by Jeremy Rifkin.[9] On the other, numerous interest groups, especially managers and attorneys who, together with couples interested in purchasing surrogates, seek to sustain the practice. We seek gentle love and nurture in life, but greed and exploitation always seem to take over.

Often only a personal drama allows for a society to come to terms with an ethical crisis. As our culture forms its new moral policy on procreation at that point where enduring values confront emerging technology, its struggle is enacted symbolically in the personal drama of two couples, Elizabeth and William Stern and Mary Beth and her now-divorced husband, Richard Whitehead.

While parents, lawyers, and lawyer-clinicians contend, in the manger at stage center is an innocent child, born amid these confused loves. The child's name is Melissa or Sara or, until secure bonds are finally designated by the courts, Baby M. The dramatis personae could have stepped out of a Sophocles tragedy.

Mary Beth Whitehead, a high school dropout toughened by bearing two children while still in her teens, was willing to incubate another new life for the lure of a ten-thousand-dollar fee. After the birth of her baby, she yearned to cling to that life to which she had now bonded and learned to love. Dr. Elizabeth Stern, a professional pediatrician at Einstein College of Medicine in New York City, delayed childbearing to finish degrees in medicine and genetics. She now suffers with a mild case of multiple sclerosis. She is married to a biochemist whose parents were killed in Nazi concentration camps. Together they now seek that filament of biologic immortality so crucial (yet so strange) to Judaism's sense of the procreative covenant, "one's own child." This child was planted by the male seed, yes, but into Mary Beth's egg, so that Judge Harvey Sorkow's ruling, giving custody to the Sterns, violated the Hebraic emphasis on the primacy of the bearing and nurturing mother and broader covenant of parental responsibility. Our "common faith" tradition, which should ground our law, is also founded on these principles.

These two couples—one marginal, the other professional; one poor, the other rich—fought for the custody of the child amid extensive newspaper and television coverage and the pressures of lawyers' fees. Should the mystery and sanctity of the transmission of life be exposed to such commercial and legal degradation? Should society formulate legislative policy that will enable or prohibit the positioning of this life-giving power within the legal or commercial apparatus? Surely our finest moral instincts lead us to believe that birth and death are sanctified mysteries and not commodities of legal and commercial definition and manipulation. The moral crisis of Western culture has been created in part because we see technological innovations as items to buy and sell in the marketplace. Parenting, baby making, fertility, and gestation are more and more seen as commodities of exchange. Suffering and dying are construed as problems to fix and fashion with technique.

The dying body, like the aborning body, is increasingly valued as a function of technological and economic activity. Our utility-based views of reality and human meaning also lead us to deal with profound human transactions, such as birth and death, sexuality and suffering, as matters of adversarial law. Since we have located such weighty issues in the legal sphere, we should not then be surprised when they become matters of calumny and contract.

With diagnostic related groups (DRGs), advertising, and legal and business exploitation gaining such influence over our decisions at life's thresholds, we will need to hold even more tenaciously to vitalistic, humanistic, and theistic values. Only thus will we honor what Tennyson has called creation's final law.[10]

HISTORICAL ETHICS

The historical is the most immediate and compelling component of ethics that speaks to the eugenic concerns we have raised. Just as the ecological vector penetrates in a special way the population issue and the epistemic the computational concerns of genetic diagnosis, so a historical perspective on ethics seems to have a natural affinity with eugenic concerns. How do recollection and remembrance ethically illumine the particular activity of eugenics and the more general body of human morality? History as morality has several meanings.

The first moral insight that history yields is that, though we sense the exhilaration of freedom, we are fundamentally and irrevocably predetermined. We cannot choose to be or not to be, although we can and do choose that for another. Though we can modify to some small extent the effect of our genetic inheritance, in the main we still have no say over our fated nature. As Karl Rahner reminds us, this fate dismays us. "The amor fati-fatum in the sense of what is uniquely committed to the individual—is no longer achieved and even this fatum is no longer accepted confidently in patience and humility as the gift of an incomprehensible love; man is subject to total neurosis."[11] The dispositions of gratitude born in gracious receipt of the life we have been given along with the initiative and ameliorative impulse that rise from our freedom lead us to seek purpose and not necessity, justice and not exploitation, altruism and not egoism.

If history is moving in a purposive direction, a historical ethic will lead us to build concrete purposes into our eugenics policies. The first step will involve alleviating those inflictions of genetic injury without harming anyone. The PKU screen and correction, if accompanied by subsequent measures to avert in-utero retardation in the babies whose mothers were corrected, provides an example of such a good policy. Indeed, morally we cannot *not* do it. Another positive value arising both from freedom and determinism would be one which purposely encourages diversity and not homogeneity. The programs of the 1920s and 1930s which sought to sterilize poor Appalachian whites and blacks and similar policies in the 1950s and 1960s which affected Texas Chicano women should always be rejected. Indeed, programs stimulating active birthing by Anglos, Asians, Amerindians, Afro-Americans, and all ethnic communities should be initiated. If measures of population constraint become necessary, they should be distributed among all groups equally.

Justice, rather than exploitation, is also a historically derived virtue. History has a leveling, equalizing effect. In the course of history, fate, luck, and circumstance favor some, but ultimately we are all born and die. In eugenics we must resist programs which divide the human family into the superior and excellent against the mediocre and inferior. A special cadre of test-tube persons possessed with superior strength and intelligence would lead us more toward a world where some few live well by taking advantage of those who are less fortunate. Eugenic spontaneity checks this regularization which leads to exploitation.

Another way to ensure justice is to enact specific policies which forbid discrimination and facilitate fair distribution. Programs for the indigent should be as rich, multifaceted, and accessible as those for the wealthy. These would include genetic counseling, parenting education, maternal care, and newborn provision. Eugenics should be a force serving the idea of justice. It does this not by discriminating and excluding but by enhancing the natural inheritance, the cultural heritage, and the environmental opportunity, allowing all to flourish.

"Service," said the black preacher, "is the rent we pay for our time here on earth." Of the historic values which enrich the human community, none is more powerful than *service and generosity.* Altruism and concern for others is a transformative force throughout history. Judiasm is steeped in human service and edification. The Christian community displaces pagan civilization precisely by virtue of its unique power of *caritas,* which prompted one outsider to observe, "See how they love one another." Karl Rahner, a leading Catholic theologian of the modern period, writes that the surest force of historical survival is not only generosity but sacrifice.

History is not made by those who try to force what is "inevitable" so that they can jump on the cart of fate in good time, but by those who are prepared to take the ultimate risk of defeat. No one can say that genetic manipulation inevitably will come. The only person who "knows" such a thing is the man who secretly wishes it to be so.

Is that kind of man a trustworthy prophet? Why should not mankind as a whole have to learn the lessons every individual has to learn in his own life if he is to survive, namely, the lessons of sacrifice and renunciation."[12]

Sacrifice and mutual service is the virtue (strength) of a person or a society that has received or achieved its own integrity. Egoism or its collective form, nationalism, arises from weakness and insecurity. The Nazi biomedical vision was posited on such felt inferiority. Adolf Hitler's eugenic ravings in *Mein Kampf* grow out of such a psychology of humiliation. "The volkish state must see to it that only the healthy beget children. . . . Here the state must act as the guardian of a millennial future. . . . It must put the most modern medical means in the service of this knowledge. It must declare unfit for propagation all who are in any way visibly sick or who have inherited a disease and can therefore pass it on."[13] Nazi eugenics indeed did attempt this diabolic ambition. Rather than symbolically drawing people and nations together in mutually edifying service, national policies now diabolically drew apart the sturdy from the wounded, the Aryan from the Jew and gypsy, the heterosexual from the homosexual.

Historic ethical insight breaks in upon the conscience through the channel of *remembrance* (*anamnēsis*). Memory can be fearful and debilitating. It can romanticize some memory and supply only irrelevant nostalgia. Creative remembrance or commemoration is the vital reliving and reenacting of moral lessons learned. Consider the ten words of the Hebrew Decalogue, for example. Most scholars suggest that these apodictic assertions are historical recitations. The command "Do not kill" may say in actuality, "You are inclined to kill; you were not meant to kill; over and again you do kill even though you should not; therefore you shall not kill." A moral imperative, in other words, emerges with the force of accrued historical experience.

Actions are founded by certain moral visions and grounded on certain constitutions. The medical art is also grounded in pivotal ethical events. The teaching of Moses, the imagination of Hippoc-rites, the ministry of Jesus, and the remembrance of Nuremberg are such nodal points of moral formation and formulation.

EUGENICS: AN ETHICAL POLICY

How do we embrace the newfound powers of eugenics within the evaluative canopy of our moral vision? Two ideologies of birth, two eugenic visions, emerge. The first picture is appearing as we slowly receive reports from China on their new national policy on birth control and population maintenance. The state has decided to exert vigorous societal control over procreation, both to sustain ad-equate population replenishment and to control overpopulation. Through a highly organized and disciplined process of indoctrina-tion, incentives, oversight, and even coercion, families are encour-aged to have one child, but no more. When a family brings a new life into this world, it is rewarded with promotion on the job and a guaranteed educational grant. These benefits are contingent upon signing a contract not to become pregnant again. Birth-control pills and careful instruction are dispensed in every commune and work-place. If a mother becomes pregnant again, disincentives are brought to bear: the job security is lost; the education grant is for-feited; abortion is proposed and, in extreme cases of resistance, is coerced.

The second picture reflects the more Horatio Alger methods of American eugenics. Peter and Kitty Carruthers won the silver medal at the Serajevo Winter Olympics (1984) with a stunning free-skating performance that dazzled even the skeptical East-bloc judges. The reports of their inauspicious beginnings intrigued people around the world. Peter and Kitty were adopted as infants from the New England Home for Little Wanderers in Boston. Their father, Charlie Carruthers, flooded their backyard and bought them cheap cardboard skates when they were five and seven years old. From those humble, unpretentious beginnings unfolded the story of ac-complishment and glory.

But today we question whether greatness can come from common origins. We have mentioned the pessimistic mentality which sees a genetic apocalypse on the horizon if we do not begin a rigorous eu-genic cleansing of the gene pool. A somewhat less cosmic version of this puritanism is found in the wish, verging on demand, found to-day as parents seek to have healthy—even perfect—children. This yearning usually has the elements of the classic eugenic visions: the desire for intelligence, physical strength, beauty, and freedom from genetic flaws which would manifest themselves as mental or physical abnormality.

This ambition to eugenerate (to change for the better) the human condition naturally expresses a deeper characteristic of the Western psyche: the desire to know the unknown, unscrew the inscrutable, avoid the deleterious, and fashion the optimal. Joseph Fletcher, who produced one of the earliest philosophical/theological treatments of human genetics, wrote, "We cannot accept the 'invisible hand' of blind chance or random nature in genetics."[14]

This underlying ideology seems to me to be a puritanism gone wild, a mania for dominion cut loose from the grace of proper humility before God and his ongoing story, a story of which we are not the final chapter. It is not surprising that this approach to nature and human nature leads us into a mentality which sees difference as disease and debility as damnation. One distinguished geneticist has argued that we should now think of genetic diseases as communicable diseases which should be brought under public quarantine control in the same way we isolate infections. When courts award damages because amniocentesis was not offered and a baby with Down's syndrome or hemophilia was born, we are obviously responding to this melioristic temper in the Western spirit gone mad.

A fitting eugenic desire, one which responds to the best eutopic and dystopic images that our moral history has established, will be hopeful but not perfectionist, just but not retaliatory, merciful but not careless. We should hope for a better chance at life for the children we bring into the world. This hope should fuel our discontent at the fact that babies still die en masse from malnourishment and are permanently stunted by maternal intoxication as a result of drug and other substance abuse. This hope should animate us to protest vigorously the ways we are polluting and poisoning our enveloping environments (air, land, water, and foods), inducing mutagenic and teratogenic births. It should prompt us to do what we can as parents and as a community to safeguard carefully those nascent lives from injury, providing the very best beginnings possible for them.

8 Legalistic Ethics of Save-or-Let-Die Decisions:

IMPERILED NEWBORNS

A few days before Christmas 1981, Jack Murphy, the 52-year-old South side Chicago bachelor, was reading the newspaper and saw a photograph and a story about a young boy who was wearing a shirt identical to one Murphy owned. The child, he read, was brain damaged, legally blind and a ward of the state. . . . For two years and nine months, Murphy drove 360 miles each week to visit Terry. He was afraid to admit to himself that he was going to adopt Terry because of the struggles he knew he would have to face. "But I couldn't let him be alone for the rest of his life. What is it like to sit in a wheelchair all of your life? That was all he knew, and he still smiled." Murphy said a verse from the Bible helped him make his decision, Mark 9, verse 36: whosoever shall receive one of such children in my name, receiveth me; and whosoever shall receive me, receiveth not me, but him that sent me.

Chicago Sun Times, **21 June 1987**

The faith and heroism of Jack Murphy brings tears to our eyes. We commend him. When Mother Teresa, Terry's godmother, touches his brow in benediction, we all vicariously confer our own blessing.

But we are not all Jack Murphys. Jack Murphy embraced an already-living, damaged, and lonely child, choosing to "father" a son many men might deny. But consider that prenatal diagnosis allows potential fathers and mothers of biologic children to glimpse a child's future—to see whether a "healthy bouncy baby" or a "burden" like Terry awaits them. Can we bear the assault to our own identity which an "imperfect" child represents? We can know now what has gone wrong in forming a baby; we can learn how to ameliorate or stabilize a "condition"; we can discuss our freedom not to treat but to let die. To anticipate that we must add to an already-strained life (one we hoped to have "redeemed" by the joy of an infant) the daily care for an imperfect being, then, furthermore, to face choosing whether or not to bear this burden—this moral responsibility is unprecedented. We bask in affluence, we cherish autonomy. Are we therefore unable to bear and share suffering such as that accompanying the birth of a defective newborn?

Before our age of medical miracles, birth came upon us quite innocently. There was very little we could do when a baby was born with its life in peril. In hushed tones, with swift acts, midwives suffocated the severely deformed newborn. The obstetrician, whose primary sense of obligation was to his patient, the mother, could put the defective child aside where it would die in silent darkness. Now bright lights and all-observant monitors of high-risk OB units and NICUs oversee the drama. A new specialty, neonatology, stands by to rescue what filament of health remains in a problem infant. Now the amnion, the tiny figure (so wrinkled and slight, yet so like us), is given voice—an advocate. Not only is the setting changed, but the dark, hidden secret of birth has become a public spectacle. The community, the law, and numerous other advocacy interest groups—Down's syndrome parents' associations, spina bifida support groups, right-to-lifers, woman's rights groups—watch closely with ideological scrutiny, some even with a genuine desire to help.

A new moral situation has taken shape as a result of this increased knowledge and enhanced therapeutic power, this more public setting for birth and the intensified and polarized moral opinions. Now a new life has come into our midst, where once all was hidden quietly inside another being, when the presentation of moral claim came solely from that host mother. In population and eugenics, even in abortion and amniocentesis, we dealt with nascent life not yet fully present to us. Now we are moving to a new level of natal ethics where a new being stands in full view before us. Once a child appears among us, a new set of affections, loyalties, rights, and obligations are activated.

Consider a set of issues generally labeled decisions of "selective nontreatment of handicapped newborns," or more recently, "the ethics of care for imperiled newborns." The very shift of language in these thematic titles reflects, as does the strange and sad saga of Baby Doe, the explosive moral intensity that charges the environment where these issues are being considered. Again, neither inflamed conviction nor cool logic helps us in resolving these agonizing clinical decisions and policies, for they require a multifaceted system of ethical analysis and wisdom.

The channel of ethical insight that we will highlight in conjunction with neonatal ethics is one which we have variously called the public, political, or legalistic. Once a community purview comes into play, we are confronted with a new normative and descriptive ethic. The normative ethic, though it shifts with public mood, is generally conservative in both senses of that word, conserving life's value and the integrity of the family. Procedurely, the social ethic is often one of minimalism and compromise. Through legislative and legal order a baseline of acceptable and unacceptable behavior is established by society. This public justice usually distills the common elements in the belief systems of all members within the pluralistic commonwealth. The process becomes one of balancing competing rights and claims—personal, professional, and public—in the context of the constitutive or charter values of that people.

In our evaluation of neonatal rescue or renunciation, we again draw on the essential genius of the ethical system under consideration. Against the backdrop of a confidence in a movement of suffering, death, and transfiguration in all that transpires in our life, we contend that, in this sphere, we should honor the primary values of patient need and physician ability, all chastened by "parental desires" and public allowance.

ETHICS AND NEONATAL ILLNESS

A limited and well-defined range of conditions constitutes the concerns of particular moral import in neonatal practice. Some babies are born with no prospect for survival: the anencephalic, for example. With others, survival is probable; there is no question about continuing treatment with all of the powers at one's disposal. Moral problems arise in a middle range of conditions, where survival is in question, prognosis questionable, and quality of life severely compromised.

Some babies are born alive but with their lives in peril because of congenital crises. These situations, where some trauma or insult has occurred during late gestation or the birth process itself, include the diabetic or drug-addicted mother, mothers with infectious diseases (e.g. rubella), complications of labor, low-birthweight infants, infants imperiled by sepsis, distress of the major organ systems, and infants with birth injuries or malformations.

Of particular concern are a group of conditions once resolved by infanticide or simple inaction which persist now because of neonatal surgery, life supports, regional centers, and transport systems. Low-birthweight infants (preemies) present some of the most difficult choices for parents and physicians and for a public that sets the ethical and economic atmosphere for the practice of medicine. Though a considerable percentage of all births occur slightly before full term, nearly 1 percent of all live births (higher among young mothers in disadvantaged communities) are extremely premature. This group is now apparently dividing into two factions—babies weighing 500–1,500 grams, and those weighing less than 500 grams. Though vulnerable to many insults, including infections, PDA (*patent ductus arteriosus*), and various metabolic disorders, these tiniest of babies are gravely imperiled because respiratory insufficiency requires intubation with the finer and smaller hardware now available. The condition often leads to intraventricular hemorrhage or bronchopulmonary dysplasia.

Preemies present a particularly difficult challenge to clinical medicine and ethics. While medical advance allows many babies to be saved, that same technology can become the vehicle of damnation because of iatrogenic injury. The more sophisticated perinatal medicine becomes and the more babies (once doomed) who now are sustained by that sophistication, the more medicine will be forced to become the cause or superintendent of their eventual death. The tragicomic drama which we have found pervading the moral essence of human existence is enacted in the preemie experience. Thus in one sense preemies are not sick; their continued life becomes their peril. Theoretically, we can push the point of viability and survivability back further and further, so that the distinction blurs between a spontaneous abortion, a miscarriage, and a premature delivery.

Other conditions which bring babies into NICUs include small gestational-age infants. These babies suffer many of the same maladies as preemies, especially physical and mental retardation. Of particular moral interest are those babies whose growth is retarded by maternal abuse (alcohol, smoking) and societal abuse (nutritional deficiency). Who is at fault? Who can help? In many of these neonatal crises we find a web of responsibility, and a wide circle of persons are involved in potential remediation.

Hyaline membrane disease (HMD) and congenital heart disease are among the major nonneurological anomalies that carry wee babies into mortal distress. If the lungs can be properly acclimatized and if the broken heart can be mended, meaningful survival is possible. This is a worthy goal, since the brain and nervous system may be intact.

Disorders such as anencephaly, microcephaly, hydrocephaly, and intraventricular intracranial bleeds present more ominous prospects. If the organ that is the seat of personality and higher consciousness is damaged, the ethics become both harder and easier. If the team decides to shunt the hydrocephalus, for example, are we redeeming a situation with good prospects, or are we stabilizing a brain that has already been severely destroyed? At this point, modern medicine, with the support of the law, must be able to initiate interventions to buy time and see what rescue is possible and then withdraw support if the news is bad. Sometimes NICU decisions are made easier when neurological deficits are known to be severe. In such cases we can let go.

But what do we do when the brain and mind are affected but not in ways incompatible with life? Perhaps the most difficult and debatable neonatal rescue decisions are those involving neural-tube defects—myelomeningocele, spina bifida systica, Down's syndrome, and the other serious chromosomal anomalies. Intelligence may be severely or only slightly damaged. Often, as in most of the tough Baby Doe decisions, the issue is forced by an anomaly secondary to the primary mental condition, say an atresia (a constricted passageway in the esophagus, stomach, or intestine). Should the presence of an operable lesion provide an opportunity to refuse treatment so that the mentally retarded baby dies? While trisomy 21 (Down's syndrome) represents a slight chromosomal malarrangement which yields a person often only slightly suboptimal, the severe cognate anomalies of trisomy 13 and 18 have such grievous presentation and prognosis that it is usually easier to decide whether to treat a secondary problem. In terms of relieving suffering, we are obligated as we are merciful not to prolong suffering in these cases.[1]

A set of questions related to our discussion of fetal research and use of abortus tissue is found in this neonatal period. Shall the organs of anencephalic babies be perfused and used for transplantation? Again the issue of redeeming a tragic circumstance appears. This play on the theme of redemption is also found in the experience of birthing and raising a Down's syndrome child. This special child, conceived in mosaic mystery, has historically been called *dinne le dia* and *geschenk gottes*, a divine gift. When Terry entered Jack Murphy's life, Jack saw the child as such a gift, a redeeming token. Often the parents of children with Down's syndrome will speak of their son or daughter as a special gift. For others it can be pure hell. The response of family, friends, neighbors, and the nation often makes the difference. In Sweden persons with Down's syndrome are given the honored position of building bicycles. In other societies, like the United States, some persons clamor to put such imperfect persons out of our way where they cannot be seen and cannot remind us of our own wounds, imperfections, and mortality. In contrast, the Special Olympics in the United States and the pilgrimages of Jean Vanier in France exemplify incorporation and affirmation.

As neonatal techniques are refined, our moral evaluation changes about what to do with babies born with these syndromes. NICUs are becoming more efficient and more accessible. The saints of the system, the specialized nurses, offer not only a masterful battery of skills but the exquisite balance of care that comes with not loving out of one's own need but in genuine concern for the baby and family. (The early experience of young women nurses whose maternal longings or aversions distorted their clinical care is now being rectified by experiential wisdom.)

Then we have the technologies. Visualization technique improves each year. The computerized cranial tomography (CCT) and nuclear magnetic resonator (NMR) technology should greatly enhance our ability to understand the condition and predict what outcome may be expected. Continuous positive airway pressure (CPAP), drugs, and surgical skills all are being refined specifically for these small and vulnerable persons.

As a result of these improvements in our capacity to know and to care, we can save and rehab more babies who should be rescued, and we can know better when our continued efforts will only intensify suffering and inflict what Engelhardt has called the "injury of prolonged existence" in a grievously debilitated state. The experience with babies born with spina bifida and Down's syndrome reflects a shift in parental, professional, and public evaluation as a result of improved capacity to care.

Twenty years ago a baby was brought to the Texas Medical Center in Houston. Her mother and her father had been referred from a small hospital in Oklahoma when she had been born with spina bifida cystica, an open exposed lesion on her spinal column. This exposed wound left her without nerve activation in the lower abdomen and hemiplegia. At that time, in the late 1960s, it was customary medical practice either to let the wound work out its lethal effect or to give the parents the option to "save or let die." These parents were given all of the known diagnostic and prognostic facts and all of the books and papers on spina bifida to read. They struggled with the difficult choice. An implantable artificial sphincter had recently been developed—a small balloon pump which could be manually inflated and deflated and miraculously restore a vital gift most of us assume, continence. While the counsel of many physicians in Great Britain and the United States at the time was not to be heroic, this family instead chose life. That the father was a clergyman and lawyer and the mother a gifted artist and teacher no doubt influenced the capacity of this family to craft a beautiful work of art out of this experience. Colleen, now an attractive young businesswoman and horse rider, grew to womanhood embraced by her family's strong love. Her mighty upper arms became strengthened by years of swinging her trunk along on her braces; she has been observed swinging herself onto a stool and, with her dexterous fingers, playing a piece on the harp.

Today, while debate about appropriate care for babies born with spina bifida continues, more nuanced selection criteria are available to make "save or let die" decisions, and because of our medical advance, we are more willing to save and rehabilitate such infants. In the future, prenatal diagnosis, the alphafeto protein sample, and the sonar scan will pick up this lesion and perhaps eliminate it completely.

Changes in the technical and social environment have also meant evaluative changes in our dealing with Down's syndrome cases. When Lejune first described the trisomy 21 anomaly, his Roman Catholic conscience warned us not to take his discovery and create a "National Institute of Death." His address before the NIH was prophetic because it presaged two decades punctuated by the Baby Doe cases, where Down's syndrome newborns with accompanying physical lesions of various sorts were delivered over by inaction or court delays to unnecessary death. Today, despite some moral self-righteousness, the right to life, the Baby Doe regulation, and the like, we do demonstrate a more responsible stewardship for these lives. For what merit is the frantic scramble to save an imperiled newborn, if we later fail to provide good lives for the afflicted but otherwise alert human beings?[2]

THE SOCIAL-POLITICAL-LEGAL ETHIC

The social, political, and legal spheres form part of the value-defining and value-transforming structure of our culture. Law and politics dominate discussions of newborn ethics, for each has played a particularly prominent role in our struggle with all that the phrase *Baby Doe* represents. The law embodies both a society's reach for a transcending sense of what is right and wrong and that instrument whereby the body politic expresses its interests. In the deepest sense of law in our culture, the judge represents both the plea of the plaintiff for justice and the divine law as the definition of justice.

In Exodus 18, Moses, the archetypal mediator of justice for our civilization, sits in judgment from dawn till dusk hearing cares brought to him by the people. His task is to judge between one and another and make them know the statutes of God and his laws (v. 16). Today, when the Indiana circuit court judge hears the case of Baby Doe or that of the "Faith Assembly" parents who refuse to bring their sick newborn in for medical care, he exerts judgment from three perspectives. He mediates the law in its codified and transcendental meaning. He also represents the society in its intention to carry out justice. Finally, he is the advocate of the accused against those who would disregard one's rights.

Baby cases are among the most difficult issues to come before the courts. Earl Shelp in *Born to Die?*[3] shows that the law, as it reflects the public interest, seeks to embody two concerns, one of which is to safeguard the integrity of the family. The state and its legal apparatus has the function of upholding the relations between spouses and between parents and children. All of the ideas of privacy, parental prerogatives, and rights in loco parentis hinge on the primacy of this sacred association. The law also affirms the rights of individuals, including children. Once a child is given a name and numbered as a citizen, he or she enjoys certain rights guaranteed by the state. Child abuse, custody law, and the recent cases of neonatal custody and forced treatment reflect this commitment.

To further explicate the ethical bearing of law on neonatal judgments, Shelp argues that "the law presumes that an adult parent has the capacity, authority and responsibility to determine what is good for one's children."[4] To presume that parents are in the best position to decide good for their children is based on the trust that parents know best and care most about their own children. When Solomon, as neonatal judge, decided to split the contested child down the middle (reminding us of the anguish of some Siamese twin surgeries), he sought to discover the genuine mother, the one who valued the child's life and well-being over her own "right." We assume parents can judge wisely concerning their children's upbringing, education, spiritual training, and discipline.

When discipline turns into punishment and punishment into abuse, society's interest in that child supersedes parental privilege, particularly when the death of a child is a possibility. If Jehovah's Witness parents decide that their leukemic child should not be transfused, the courts will most often step in, declare temporary custody, and order treatment. In neonatal cases the courts will sometimes overrule parents, as with the Danville Siamese twins and round 1 of Baby Jane Doe. In other cases, the courts support parental decisions, as in Baby Doe and the Baby Jane Doe appellate decision.

In public policy, legislation, and public-health measures, society also exerts its values concerning neonates. Regional perinatal care centers in Canada and then the United States have been established, and laws enacted. The state of Colorado until very recently had a law which required unwed mothers to nurse their babies. Safe milk laws, regulations for reporting premature births, and state and national programs to fund perinatal care all reflect two values: to minimize perinatal injury and to enhance opportunities for a better life. As a result of these efforts, neonatal mortality has drastically decreased over the last two decades.

Our political ethics seek to absorb some of the pain of life into the body of the family and the body politic. The family is seen as a buffer against the traumas of life. The societal body, too, can absorb pain and injury and minimize the burst of life's pains.

THE JURISPRUDENTIAL ESSENCE OF ETHICS

Three themes of legalistic parlance come into play in neonatal and all medical ethics. These themes are derived from our religious and moral heritage.

Life. The Baby Doe cases have occurred at a moment in political history characterized by a significant societal value shift. We live in a day of reassertion of a "right to life" public philosophy. Our law-making leadership has considered a "life begins at conception" clarification of the Fourteenth Amendment. Phyllis Schlafly has promulgated a view on family life and woman's destiny that has gained such wide currency as to stymie the passage of the Equal Rights Amendment. The Reagan Administration has declared itself opposed to abortion and the *Roe* v. *Wade* Supreme Court decision and pressed Baby Doe and Baby Jane Doe guidelines. Dr. Everett Koop, a Philadelphia pediatrician and surgeon general of the United States, had for years expressed a right-to-life, antiabortion message in the context of the broader theme of historic catastrophe and decline of the Christian West. His films (made with colleague-pastor Francis Schaeffer) detailing the plight of the human race are known to millions. Koop, like Dr. William Kieswetter of Pittsburgh's Children's Hospital, is a distinguished surgeon with experience with Siamese twins. These men share an evangelical-fundamentalist theological persuasion. Dr. Koop has expressed grave reservations about the probity of neonatal antidysthanasia (allowing defective newborns to die). This becomes clear in his responses to the Hopkins Down's syndrome case and the Duff and Campbell review of Yale University cases where children with severe defects were allowed to die.[5]

As we ponder the theme of defending life, it might be proposed that the birth of severely deformed children insults and assaults the lives of families and that self-defense is justifiable. Although this notion must be pursued with utmost care, it seems relevant to the discussion. In contrast to the dominant theme of new life as divine blessing, there is in Jewish ethics a thread that sees the fetus, particularly the distorted fetus, as an aggressor against the life of the mother.[6] Roman Catholic medicomorality has also pondered the case of the baby whose birth demands the death or injury of its mother.[7] Whether the right to life refers also to the vitality and viability of a family remains a crucial issue to consider.

In the Danville Siamese twin case, the right-to-life issue was raised. Many persons in medicine, nursing, philosophy, theology, and ethics felt that the initial decision of doctors and family not to begin life-support—even feeding and hydration—was justifiable in light of the jeopardy the birth presented to the family and the drawn-out suffering it implied for the children. Joseph Fletcher, whose writings on genetics, abortion, and care of defective newborns are widely known,[8] felt that withholding treatment could be justified on the basis of the overriding harmful effects on the family and on many persons if the lives were prolonged. In sheer ethico-metrics, the costs greatly outweighed the benefits.

Alternatively, Paul Ramsey argued that it was wrong not to feed and hydrate such newborns. The principle of the covenant of life with life mandated support, although he found extraordinary mea-sures (e.g. resuscitation) questionable. A critical determination for Ramsey was whether or not the twins were dying. Could they be separated? Could one be saved? The answer to those questions would determine the moral status of particular life-saving or death-hastening actions. Ramsey also felt that the ultimate legal adjudica-tion of the case should occur at two levels. One proceeding should render a decision on the issue of euthanasia. Another deliberation should consider penalties.

Willard Gaylin, John Fletcher, and others regretted that this case ever moved into the public arena. It should have been handled in the confidentiality of the family–medical team relationship, with consultation of an ethics committee and with collegial discussion in order to develop clear, unequivocal decisions to which all persons involved were party and agreed. Consensus should have been sought. In the face of moral uncertainty and lacking consensus, sus-taining life is a community obligation, and the right to life as per-sonal entitlement must be preeminent. This stance, supporting Ramsey's, seems one in keeping with values of mercy and probity.

Liberty. Next to the value of life, the most widely invoked topic in medical ethics today is liberty. Gerald Dworkin, Mark Siegler, and many others have used the criteria of freedom, self-determination, and parental prerogatives to clarify moral judgment.[9] To whom does the decision to prolong or protract the life of these children belong? Do the parents, the physicians, the state, or the courts have juris-diction? We commit most decisions about procreation and family life to the parents. Or, better stated, we challenge and usurp the oversight of the family only in situations of obvious neglect, abuse, or brutality. Otherwise, what Judge Bork calls the "general assump-tion of freedom" prevails. Does this case belong under the rubric "right to privacy" (a derivative of liberty), or is it a concern of com-munity justice?

Parental authority is a theme that supports the view that the Danville case should never have passed into the public domain. The decision, admittedly profound and tragic, should have transpired in the privacy, confidentiality, and discretion of the parent-physician relationship. The blunders of communication or quandaries of conscience that drew it into the public limelight are understandable and forgivable, but as one legal colleague has said, "This should not go into the courts; they have no superior wisdom to adjudicate these searching questions. Bad cases—bad law."

Happiness. The final theme that has been helpful in pondering the Danville case is happiness—but not the banal superficial notion of comfort and complacency which we currently label happiness. The deeper meanings of felicity, compassion, justice, and blessedness of which the Beatitudes speak bear strongly on this case. Vatican radio, condemning newborn euthanasia, which "distinguishes between lives which have meaning because they are useful, efficient and joyous and those to which all meaning has been denied because they are judged useless, inefficient and without joy," questioned our common ways of determining the "value" of a child's life.[10]

Happiness is not a facile matter of delights and a sense of usefulness; rather, it is fulfillment that becomes possible in an environment of caring. What does this mean for parents who in care have drawn away and begun to grieve both the disappointment and the loss of this, their only offering of ongoing life to this world, their own flesh and blood? What does it mean to demand that they now remain attached, or worse yet, that they are not to be entrusted with this offspring? The Danville parents regained custody of the children, but the possibility of court intervention threatened the family.

Family, the basic covenant of life, is the care-giving and life-giving fabric that patterns, binds, and weaves each of us into a history and a future. It is the paradigm for and the representation of the divine embrace of our life. It is only within covenants of care, where happiness is a prospect because hope, not despair, prevails, that life and liberty are possible. Where children are unwanted and neglected and no nurture is present, only frustration and violence are possible. If we acknowledged this fact, perhaps we would not magnify this and other singular cases out of proportion but might begin to work on the real childhood moral crises of our society such as the starvation death of children en masse around the world and the fact that, even in America, a major cause of retardation is maternal and infant malnutrition and that 40 percent of children born in Chicago do not have legal or otherwise accountable fathers. If human happiness and well-being are to flourish, we must reactivate the intimate communities of caring such as the churches and neighborhoods and thus relieve the public agencies, which should be expected to serve only those for whom no other help is possible.

Vitality, liberty, and felicity are noble public values which can sustain us through these thorny and troublesome issues.

A PUBLIC ETHIC

As we witness the deeply divisive nature of such issues as abortion or newborn euthanasia, it becomes clear not only that we need a thoughtful public ethic, convincing in both its substantive and procedural aspects, but that we need to secure for that public ethic pastoral and transcendental insight. For that reason we need to return to an earlier suggestion that our society adopt both an ethic that is "deep"' and "surface," both "background" and "foreground," and that we develop mechanisms by which the one enriches the other. The closest proposal we have for such a cooperative public ethic, one which intermingles reflective elements of deep belief and minimalist procedural legalities, is found in Tristram Engelhardt's provocative book *The Foundations of Bioethics*.

What shall such a two-tiered policy ethic look like, and how shall it address neonatal save-or-let-die decisions? Let us explore the following thesis: while a tolerant and pluralistic society cannot implement any parochial belief or value system, no matter how majoral or consensual it has become, that society cannot violate the precepts of that particular or common faith. Rather, a society should seek to affirm positive value and to restrain, within the limits of appropriate freedom, the injury persons do toward themselves and to others. Such a public policy will *inhibit* harm, *tolerate* diversity of conscience and belief, and *facilitate* the emergence of salutary values and practices.

Present Baby Doe legislation effectively *inhibits* overly cavalier and thoughtless practices of allowing newborns to die simply because they are not perfect. The present policy, focused in state statute rather than strong-armed national surveillance and control, holds that ordinary treatment must not be withheld from imperiled or handicapped newborns unless (1) the treatments are futile in the sense that they prolong suffering without offering healing or cure and (2) death is imminent and unavoidable. Based on the doctrine of "right to life" and the inviolable sacredness of a person's existence, this policy wisely inhibits too-easy decisions to allow a defective newborn to die.

The emphasis on local decision making involving physicians and family and the health-care team expresses a social policy of *tol-*

erating diversity of conscience and variation in the pain-bearing capacity that different families possess. A child may be born with a short-gut syndrome and be unable to survive without permanent and perpetual technical infusion of nutrition. Babies like David who are born with severe combined immunologic deficiency and require lifelong care in a germ-free bubble may be treated in a similar manner. Since these illnesses are incompatible with life and the intervention will not cure but rather prolong the terminal process, parents may in certain circumstances choose not to continue treatment. The casuistic wisdom, looking back over a long series of Baby Doe cases, has brought case law to the same point.

Finally, the emphasis on teaching ethics in home and school, as well as in church, synagogue, and professional school, calls attention to the need to *facilitate* positively the salutary values we wish to instill. Infant Care Review Committees (ICRCs) and Pediatric Bioethics Committees are now actively working in most hospitals and medical centers sponsoring educational conferences for medical professionals and the public on the substantive ethical principles and the procedural practices at stake in neonatal decision making. Active parent support groups also help to shoulder burdens and to encourage cosufferers.

A common-sense wisdom now seems to be emerging about when to save and when to let die. Armed with more precise epistemic data, especially diagnostic and prognostic data, encouraged by clearer convictions about life's worth and the ability we have to care and help one another to care, we are arriving at something like Aristotle's golden mean between vices. There was a vicious quality to the too easy abandonment of the sick, deformed, and retarded in antiquity and in the early modern era. As Callahan states, the value of sanctity of life is such a newfound and unprecedented human conviction that we need safeguard it, since it has been with us such a short time. Let us consider some special issues of neonatal ethics in the light of the moral position we have espoused.

SPECIAL ISSUES IN NEONATAL ETHICS

Four moral proposals to deal with the issue of imperfect and imperiled newborns have been made which focus their suggestion on the specific leitmotif of our study—the analysis and absorption of pain and suffering. Let us discuss the proposal of Joseph Fletcher and others that a scale of severity and morbidity be drawn to determine who shall live and who shall die. Then we look at the thought of pediatrician-ethicist William Bartholome of the University of Kansas. Bartholome proposes that delicate calculations of morbidity and mortality be drawn so that we discern clearly when we are dealing with a living or a dying child. Third, we consider Paul Ramsey's proposal of transferring and sharing the burden of the child who presents acute need throughout the covenanting community. Finally, we discuss the question of social policy as the body politic chooses by its programmatic whether to increase or decrease the incidence of premature births.

Joseph Fletcher has proposed in numerous unpublished papers and speeches that we develop a scale of severity to ground medical policy for babies born with genetic defects. At one end of the spectrum a moral policy of palliative care alone is proposed for babies born with conditions like Tay-Sachs disease, Lesch-Nayan syndrome, trisomy 13 and 18, severe malignancy at birth, and anencephaly and microcephaly. Less severe but still grave disorders call for supportive care (such as feeding and antibiotics) but not corrective surgery or heroic curative efforts. Down's syndrome infants with serious anomalies and other neural-tube defects would fall into this group. Finally, in a group of milder syndromes and conditions, intense treatment and efforts to stabilize and correct anomalies is called for.

Fletcher's moral calculus is based on two ideas. First, there is an assessment of neurological viability, intellectual power, and humanhood. If the foundations for personality development and intellectual activity (memory, IQ, etc.) is missing, the obligation to save and sustain is removed. Fletcher does not distinguish, as Engelhardt has done, between persons and nonpersons but simply argues that claim and obligation is diminished when the brain is damaged. A second theme in Fletcher's moral reflection is the requirement of a "love ethic." The essence of Fletcher's ethical conviction is rooted in compassion. Great burdens which crush one's spirit, take one to the verge of breakdown, devastate marriages, decimate savings, and otherwise challenge the family's well-being need not be undertaken. On this point Fletcher concurs with the classic Roman Catholic position on obligation in "extraordinary" circumstance. The deformed child can be let go, the tragedy accepted, the family can move on, perhaps to try again for a healthy baby. A theology or philosophy based on relief of pain and nonimposition of suffering runs through Fletcher's thought, informing his views on terminal care, death, and dying, even issues of war and peace. The central force in his ethic is the agapic ethic that the Christian gospel has found to be the most powerful reality in the world.

We commend Fletcher for the spirit of kindness and understanding in his ethics. The only critique we would offer on the compassion side of his neonatal ethic is that it asks of parents too little by way of courage and patience. The heart of the agapic ethic in its biblical setting is sacrificial love. Fletcher's love ethic plays too much into the hands of our comfort-seeking, challenge-shirking ethos. The more telling critique of his neonatal approach is leveled against the "normalcy" doctrine. The critique we offer is the same which is directed toward utilitarian ethics in general. The emphasis on quantification of benefits and risks is too arbitrary, as is the reduction of human value to the measurable criteria of humanhood. The mystery of the human person and the unpredictable depths of human capacity should lead us to remain open to receiving the graces of life and parenthood. A multifaceted ethic often repudiates the imperative that might arise from any single channel of moral insight. The singular claim of householding, impulse, instinct, feeling, principle, calculation, law, memory, belief, or even hope is sometimes confounded by the cooperative, comprehensive ethical perspective. Bereft of any compelling intuition, one must struggle along into the unknown without any answer. Ironically, this course itself, not acting at all because of lack of clear direction, may embody wisdom.

William Bartholome is known through the country as the pediatrician on service at Johns Hopkins University when the first chronicled Baby Doe case occurred in 1971. In this celebrated case, the parents of a Down's syndrome baby with duodenal atresia refused an operative permit, condemning the baby to a death after fifteen agonizing days of starvation. The reenacting of this case has been seen by millions of people in the film *Who Shall Survive?* It has also provided the point of departure for many articles and commentaries on neonatal ethics. Drawing on traditional medical wisdom, which apprehends in the patient what are called "the signs of Hippocrates," and honoring both pagan and biblical wisdom, which finds it evil either to treat the living as if they were dying or the dying as if they were living, Bartholome asks an extensive battery of diagnostic and prognostic questions about the trajectory of the new life. Combined sympathies for the imperiled child and the anguished parents lead him to see ethics, not so much as a process of discovering the "right" answer, but as one of struggle—lost in a fog, abandoned in a forest, bewildered and desperate for some light, a leading hand, a way out.

In my own clinical experience, there is moral legitimacy in the effort to discern through careful diagnostics and prognostics where the life is tending. This can lead us with wonder not to assault the terrible but blessed markings of death's approach. Paul Ramsey raised the same issue when he asked in the case of the Danville Siamese twins whether they were living or dying and whether therapy was sustaining or safeguarding life or prolonging dying.

Bartholome's reflection in the aftermath of the Hopkins case has concluded that a wrong was done to let that baby die. The many parents who came forward after the case expressing their willingness to adopt such a child have led him in subsequent cases to seek ways to share the initial shock and trauma with parents in more sensitive ways, to find others to come to the aid of the frightened parents (e.g. Down's syndrome support groups), and in last resort to suggest that adoptive parents might come to take on vicariously the burden that is too great for the natural parents to bear. Bartholome, for example, supported the final decision in the Becker case, where, when the natural parents refused coronary surgery for their Down's syndrome son and neglected visiting him, the court awarded custody to another couple who for many years had cared and looked after him. As I look back over the twenty years of my own clinical ethics consultation, when physicians, nurses, or parents invite me to share their ordeal, I usually ask them to ponder whether their baby is struggling to live or struggling to die. Often a forceful and comforting conviction about what to do becomes clear once that question is considered.

Deeply ingrained in the physician's oath is the injunction that one never use the art to harm another. The Hippocratic dictum *primum non nocere* and the signs of Hippocrates as signals to withdraw are not so much gestures of abandonment as they are recognition of the force of disease, the frightful power of medicine, and the ultimate concession to destiny and transcendence. Medicine's power must be unleashed only in the service of life and health (*natura naturans*), never in an assault on death and never for its own intrigue. Bartholome's ethic captures the essence of this wisdom.

By way of critique, we might suggest that, if Fletcher overemphasizes parental suffering to the point of indulgence, Bartholome overromanticizes child suffering and in the process downplays parental anguish and conscience. Fetal and neonatal pain and suffering, though surely agonizing and pitiful, exist in a different order than adult suffering. Adults bring both history and anticipation to their experience of pain. What we know about the neurology of neo-natal pain and analgesic response make it inappropriate to over-value it when balanced against hurt to parents.

Paul Ramsey spares no words in his critique of the parental care and convenience which entails lethal neglect of newborns. Like Bartholome, he stops short of labeling neonaticide murder and rather calls it injustice: "To deliberately make medical care a function of inequities that exist at birth is evidently to add injustice to injury and fate."[11] When we claim that newborns should be allowed to die because a marriage is fragile or a family is poor, we create an unconscionable injustice.

The argument for equality and for treating all cases alike is specious. It covers the basic point that Ramsey and Bartholome wish to make for the sacred inviolability of the newborn child. Justice as equality is an abstract doctrine that is more superficial than the rigorous ethics of these two scholars. The argument, I believe, is presented in the same way in which the American Academy of Pediatrics presents the privacy-of-practice argument on the Baby Doe case. The argument appeals to conservative political administrations, but the privacy of physician-patient practice has never been strongly emphasized by the progressive voices in the American Academy.

The academy's proposal of absorption and displacement of suffering, however, does deserve careful attention. In the same way that Bartholome, recollecting the Hopkins case, wished for options of adoption, Ramsey quotes with favor Dr. Chester A. Swimyard. When dealing with shocked parents who must make save-or-let-die decisions, Dr. Swimyard takes as a strategy a class separation between what the child needs by way of immediate care, what will happen later, and who will look after the long-range needs of the child. Assuming that Dr. Swimyard is able to set aside his vested interests as a rehabilitationist, we can find some merit in this approach. We desperately need mechanisms for the community to say to distressed parents, "You are not alone; we intend to go through this with you." There is also an acute need for the society that voices a pro-life ethic in abortion and neonatal decisions to follow through with impressive systems of subsidy, institutional care, rehabilitation, and rigorous programs to develop the potentials of those human beings whose lives we have saved. Absorption, sharing, and resourcing one another through suffering are fundamental imperatives of justice and beneficence in today's world.

Perhaps the cruelest sequel to the moral hypocrisy of saving, then damning in neglect, is (1) the crisis of postnatal mortality and

(2) the scandal of socially engineered prematurity rates. Low-birthweight infants are born in rates that correspond directly to social policies of maternal and child care. When monies are cut back, the birth of preemies accelerates, as does the cost of neonatal intensive care. Some years ago the parishes around New Orleans committed themselves, with the aid of state and national funding, to reduce the birthrate of premature infants. An American version of the Chinese "barefoot physician" program was adopted. Older women who, though not necessarily well educated, were street-wise, were put on small salaries and trained extensively to visit all of the shanties and housing projects where pregnant girls were living. They taught these childbearing children how to care for themselves and their babies. These future mothers were given not only information but tangible aid to provide adequate nutrition and other critical needs. When the program's effects were felt, a dramatic reduction of preemie and other imperiled births was recorded. All went well until in the early 1980s these funds were cut, along with those of most other community-based welfare efforts. Premature births, infant mortality, and all the other salutary indices of health shot up again. It seems we prefer to pay the high cost of NICUs rather than address the source of the problem.

Our ethical system offers an insight into the cause of this stupidity and moral hypocrisy. We are simultaneously a society of life-saving heroics and subsequent contempt toward children. We have a strong pro-life "save the defective newborns" ethos, followed by policies of neglect for those we have saved. Our pathos-probing ethic would answer this duplicity in the great residue of guilt for the careless way we have sacrificed child life for centuries and especially in recent years. Children die of starvation in Ethiopia and the sub-Sahara. Children were sacrificed in large numbers in the war in Vietnam. Today we casually sacrifice millions of children each year by abortion, malnourishment, child abuse, and neglect. Our residue of guilt in the face of this infanticide prompts us, I would contend, to verbal gestures of respect and advocacy, but an esteem that is only nominal and verbal, because it is not followed by concrete actions.

If we look into our moral soul, we will see a serious ethical ambivalence regarding newborns. If we resort to political and legal-moral insights, we will establish a bedrock of foundational values. But we confront a moral crisis of the human spirit. We must therefore evaluate our moral consideration again to the level of transcendental reference.

9 Theological Ethics of Graceful Release:

LIFE-THREATENING ILLNESS AND DEATH IN CHILDREN

Whoever receives a child in my name receives me.

Matt. 18:5

The people brought little children to him, that he would lay hands on them and pray but the disciples rebuked them. "Allow the little children to come to me, do not forbid them," he said, "of such is the kingdom of heaven."

Matt. 19:13–14

It was one of the most remarkable operations ever performed. The twenty-two-hour marathon ended at 5:15 A.M. A seventy-member medical team had culminated five months' preparation and separated seven-month-old Siamese-twin boys who were born joined at the head. Patrick and Benjamin Binder, born on February 2 to Josef and Teresa Binder of Ulm, West Germany, were attached at the back of the head, sharing a large area of skull, brain tissue, and the sagittal superior sinus, the main vein which drains blood and fluids from the brain.

During the surgery the skull was opened and the brain tissue

149

exposed. Some of the pericardial tissue that encases the heart was removed to construct new veins and sinuses for the babies' heads. The bodies were cooled to a hypothermic state of 68 degrees Fahrenheit, their blood was drained, and they were kept in "suspended animation" with stopped heart and near-silent metabolism during the operation. After the operation they were kept in a drug-induced coma in order to prevent swelling. Although prospects of recovery were no better than 50 percent, doctors said that without the operation they had no real potential for a normal life. "They would have had to remain bed-ridden and relegated to lying on their backs for as long as they lived."[1]

The courageous suffering of the children, the desperate faith and trust of the parents, and the heroic efforts of the medical team, though astounding, are not the primary impressions one reaches from this case. More impressive, is the enormous investment of energy expended in the small chance of rescuing these children from what was perceived to be an intolerable life of suffering and constrained life-style. Ever since Chang and Eng were born in Siam in 1811 and displayed here and abroad by Barnum, our age of autonomy and enlightenment cannot bear the thought of persons being so symbiotically conjoined. Even though our perceptions are not those of the children, who, let us remember, know no other reality than the existence they now have, we feel that even death is to be preferred to such contorted existence. In this perception and value we have proceeded in this past century to attempt to separate and in most cases kill, albeit the merciful death of anesthesia, most Siamese children.

In this chapter we consider the plight of little children suffering with life-threatening conditions and those facing death. We consider our perceptions of value as in the role of parents, professionals, or the public as we look upon this plight. Two Gospel texts commend to us the responsibilities of both endearment and relinquishment when it comes to the "little children" (Matt. 18:5, 19:13–14). All parents who raise children know the exquisite balance necessary between holding near and letting go. This moral dialectic is commended to us most clearly by the theological vector of ethics. In theology we confront the dialectical reality of life here and life beyond, of time and eternity, nature and supernature, the world and God. This dialectic forms the basis for both respectful receipt and reverential relinquishment of our own life and that of a child.

Theology is also the art of ecstasis, being moved beyond ourselves, standing outside of ourselves. Our moral and ethical life has much to do with establishing a perspective which transcends ourselves, putting ourselves as much as is possible inside the experience of another. What does that person feel? How much pain is this baby feeling? What would Karen Quinlan want done if she could speak to us? All of these questions point toward the essence of the universal moral imperative embodied in the ethics which mandates, "Do unto others as you would have them do unto you," and in Immanuel Kant's dictum, "Act so that that which you do could always and everywhere be done."

Placing one's head and heart inside a member of one's own family or a loved one is particularly difficult. When Joseph Quinlan, Karen's stepfather, was being evaluated as to whether he had her best interest "in mind," the court considered both the difficulty and the strength of being her adoptive father. The peculiar blend of endearment and estrangement that is found between siblings or parents and children creates an ambivalent situation when it comes to judging what is in the other's best interest. This is especially true when it comes to mother or father with a child, especially a very small child, who has not yet begun its work of self-identification and separation. A child is a mirror of ourselves. A little baby mirrors our past, present, and future. The child draws into view our genetic past and what we had been as children. The reminder is usually humiliating. The child in some sense portrays us to the world and to ourselves. The child is also our gift to the future of the world—some would say, our immortality. In the light of this complexity, it may be asked how reliable the judgment of a parent is of what is in the mind of the child or what is best for the child. Unless it be the deranged Richard III ("the sons of Edward sleep in Abraham's bosom") or abusing parents, the fact is that most parents cannot bear to see their children suffer. The practice of kidnapping or threatening harm to a child in order to extract anything from a parent attests to this fact. This theme of harm and death to one's beloved, of course, becomes the center of theological insight in the biblical tradition, as Kierkegaard highlighted in his treatment of Abraham's sacrifice of his son Isaac. Think of the crucifixion—"God loved the world so much that he gave his only Son" (John 3:16 NEB). Putting children forth into the world is a crucifixion of self—in this case, the selves we call parents. This forthgiving entails suffering, death, and transfiguration. Through new life we yield our life over to death and therein find life anew.

Children are momentarily given over to us in order that we in turn may give them over. One nurse brought a newborn baby to the hospital room where the parents waited and said, "Here she is—hold her for a while." To hold a child "for a while" is all we can ever hope for. While the prophet can see through the veil of suffering to what lies beyond, such insight remains beyond the ken of ordinary mortals.

Our protective embrace of a child can be both saving and damning. Mothering can become smothering; fathering, paternalizing. On one neonatal unit recently a very committed and concerned father (who was also a computer scientist) wanted to monitor and record every action on his child—the light, heat, noises, medication, procedures—working them all into a computer program. Needless to say, his oversight became damaging to the baby.

Often we have to hand over the well-being of our child to another. Jan Van Eys, the head of pediatrics at the M. D. Anderson Cancer Hospital in Houston, evokes the biblical image of Elijah with the widow of Zarephath to show the relinquishment that is required for revival. The woman's son had collapsed in cardiopulmonary arrest, and "the spirit had left him."

> "Give me your son," [Elijah] said. He took the boy from her arms and carried him up to the roof-chamber where his lodging was, and laid him on his own bed. . . . "O Lord my God, is this thy care for the widow with whom I lodge, that thou has been so cruel to her son?" Then he breathed deeply upon the child three times and called on the Lord, "O Lord my God, let the breath of life, I pray, return to the body of this child." The Lord listened to Elijah's cry, and the breath of life returned to the child's body, and he revived; Elijah lifted him up and took him down from the roof into the house, gave him to his mother and said, "Look, your son is alive." Then she said to Elijah, "Now I know for certain that you are a man of God and that the word of the Lord on your lips is truth." (1 Kings 17:19–24 NEB).

In this classic text of CPR, the resuscitation or resurrection is placed within the context of unjust affliction. This young child should not have arrested suddenly. Some wrong had crossed the widow mother's path. The case may even have been her new boarder himself, Elijah. Similarly, life-threatening disease or death in a child is enigmatic suffering: "Why is this happening?" Van Eys continues: "The affliction of cancer is an unacceptable assault on the helpless and innocent child, one that the parents cannot allow. The child has been stricken in an unjust way, and the parents are certain they can rectify the injustice. They hope that, like Elijah, the physician can restore life to their child."[2]

Suffering cries out for justice and as such is a moral reality. Justice brings rectification or *explanation* to suffering. Explanation here means the laying out on a table, making plain, showing its pattern, its layout, its meaning. Not only does the child's desperate need demand the taking up of this suffering, the healer's power also creates a moral demand.

The young girl was in her early teens. She had become sick with an hepatic infection of unknown etiology, perhaps a virus infection. In any case, she lay in a stage 3, deep hepatic coma. The liver-transplant team swung into action. One of the team flew by chartered airplane to secure an organ from a distant city. The operation took all night. The next day, like the dead child in the Gospels, the young girl sat up. Her eyes opened, she spoke, she was alive again. The "don't just do something—stand there" ethic is intolerable in the face of life-threatening need and possible life-saving power.

NEWBORN DISEASE AND DEATH

We come into this world possessed of survival potential amid extreme vulnerability. At birth the skull plates are still soft and unmended but falls on the head surprisingly do as little damage as did the tight squeeze out of the birth canal. We are protected by maternal immunities so powerful that even a lethal disease like SCID is masked for months until the mother's defensive strength passes and an inborn vulnerability is expressed. But the baby is also extremely dependent and vulnerable. Without the breast or bottle it shrivels and dies in a few weeks. Parents down through the ages have knelt by the crib and prayed with little ones, "If I should die before I wake. . . . " This was not morbid piety but a realistic reckoning that an infection, arrest, or some other sort of crib death might occur before morning. Until recent decades almost all family histories are marred with the death of one or more children.

One of the sudden and frightening ways that babies are swept away is crib death, technically called sudden infant death syndrome (SIDS). In the United States each year nearly ten thousand babies, usually under six months of age, die in their sleep. A thief in the night, like sudden coronary death in adults, this shock comes to one of every five hundred newborns. In 15 percent of the cases autopsy reveals some structural anomaly in the cardiovascular or central nervous system or an overwhelming infection. In the other 85 percent of cases, there seems to be a "final common pathway" in which a violent laryngospasm occurs, and breath is dramatically wrenched or drawn away from the little body.

I use the phrase "drawn away," not to deny a mechanical event of some kind, but to call into question the reductionist mechanical explanation. I was once asked to offer ethics consultation on a research protocol which sought to identify adults who were thought to be vulnerable to sudden coronary death because of certain profiles. The idea of the experiment was to put monitors on some of these parameters (e.g. sudden decrease of venous pressure), then shock the person awake at night when any one of these suspicious physical events occurred. I was excused from the project when I raised the question as to what was wrong with dying suddenly in one's sleep at the end of a good life.[3]

Like sudden coronary death, SIDS also is no longer acceded to as "giving up the spirit" or the divine expiration of our breath. It is now a syndrome we wish to understand and conquer, perhaps even to the point of keeping the baby perpetually awake. I know another baby who was born with the severe injuries of a Siamese birth who had to be suctioned for secretions every thirty minutes, day and night, every day of its short four-year life. SIDS parents are grief stricken and guilt ridden. They feel something deeply unjust has been done to them and that they, in some self-recriminating way, must be to blame—that they, too, should have sat up all night guarding against death. This complex of suffering is not helped at all when the police and child-welfare investigators show up asking questions.

Grief and guilt lift the experience of loss of a baby to SIDS into the realm of moral concern. Grief is the experience of being undeservedly abandoned both by the deceased and by those who ought to offer support. Suffering *ought* not to be borne alone. The ethical doctrine of compassion that we have propounded in this book contends that our vocation is to suffer for and with others. The baby with SIDS in some mysterious way dies for the sins of the world and into the grace of God. How might this be? Since the incidence of SIDS deaths across the years is constant, it might be the case that this division bears a certain portion of the weight of genetic load and congenital accident on behalf of the human race. In this sense perinatal devastations can be seen as part of the burden of evil that must be borne and absorbed by someone. SIDS may also be the consequence of some human malice or neglect. This could be anything from environmental toxification to some absence of sympathetic identification. We die daily and kill daily. That also is part of the sin that we have let loose in the cosmos.

Finally, it is important that the counseling sessions that follow the death in the first months of bereavement raise the concern of giving birth to other children. Our perceptions about why this happened, what it means, and where we go from here are moral perceptions which affect how we believe and act toward ourselves and toward others. The sick and dying stand as a judgment before us. Some are able to identify with such persons and are saved. Others are lost.

Death into the grace of God is the transfigurative culmination of the drama of redemption. Dostoyevsky said the death of a child was sufficient reason to doubt God's existence. But why is the death of a tiny child any more absurd than the death of a teenager in a motorcycle accident or a young mother to breast cancer or an old man to congestive heart failure? Each life is complete in itself. Each story is finished, at least in this episode. To avoid the two shoals of shipwreck—unbounded aggression and debilitating apathy—our perceptions ought to prompt us to the delicate equipoise of resistance and resignation of which Teilhard spoke: "We must struggle against death with all our force, for it is our fundamental duty as living creatures. But when, by virtue of a state of things (transitory, no doubt, but inevitably linked to the state of growth of the world), death takes us, we must experience that paroxysm of faith in life that causes us to abandon ourselves to death as to a falling into a greater life."[4]

Our children are taken from us by one cause or another. If it is not war, starvation, or plague amid adversity, it is cancer, SIDS, and accidents amid affluence. Any way they are taken is cruel and unjust, and we are left brokenhearted. At the extreme end of this horror is the children's home in the town of Adieu, France.[5] In this orphanage Jewish children were provided a kind and happy home until Klaus Barbie had them deported to the death camp. When joined to the waste of war and insurgency, kidnapping and neglect, this kind of malevolent infanticide lays a very heavy burden of guilt on the moral soul of modern humanity. This guilt shapes in part the remorse, resistance, and resignation that we have toward the other vectors of child morbidity and mortality. We perceive serious disease and death in children with blame, denial, disavowal, even irrational therapeutic aggression—all out of this residue of shame in our individual and collective moral psyche.

We seem to be able to do very little to combat SIDS and accidents and even less about war, hunger, and deprivation. So cancer becomes a zone of possible advance, even conquest, and therefore receives an enormous energy to vanquish the enemy. Acronyms for the multimodal cancer therapies, assaults like MOP and WHOP, sound like code words for military operations. In these first three decades of antineoplastic and cytotoxic drugs and multimodal therapies, the aftermath has sometimes been celebrated victory, sometimes a burned-out war zone.

Again we must be reminded that it is very difficult to identify with children suffering from cancer, especially little babies. We may too easily decide that a child would not want to go through the struggle to arrest and reverse serious disease, especially when his or her body is the war zone that will be cut, poisoned, and scorched. On the child's behalf we may find the nausea, hair loss, brain damage, and sterility too much to bear. We may even use Golden Rule reasoning—"I wouldn't want to go through that myself." On the other hand, our perceptions may too easily brush off discomfort and injury. With children, when we must make the decisions, we become so accustomed to the "growing pains" that children must face in the normal course of life that we do not hesitate to add some new burdens. Too often parents blithely concede to what "is always done" when one has Hodgkins lymphoma, leukemia, or osteosarcoma. We blithely assume that it is just another routine ordeal to be borne in the game of life. This concession to what is thought to be custom has often superseded the hard choices of sound rational decision. The perception that one does what is expected is treacherously enforced by a medical ethos which joins the concept of natural history of disease with "treatment of choice" mythology and unconsciously and implicitly claims that "this is the thing to do." One of the hard-gained but terribly important contributions of the cancer research centers these recent decades has been to remind families that rote decisions are facile and dangerous. In the years ahead, the great centers of novel and investigative therapy will have the moral obligation not only to find good and safe treatments but to help parents hone these considered perceptions and judgments about whether or not to treat, about choosing between treatment A and B with X morbidity and Y mortality, about when to begin and when to stop.

When we are the surrogate or agent for another, as in the case of parents with very small children, spiritually astute perceptions are required. This means that they must be ecstatic (standing outside of oneself) and intuitive. Our decisions based on those perceptions must be trustworthy to the one in whose place we stand and faithful in the sense of participating in those realities which are larger and ultimate. We see now the indispensability of a theological dimension to ethics.

Another insight about human perception contributes to ethics and clinical judgment. This little child does not believe in the reality or finality of death. In his innocence, the child perceives the truth behind the contrary apparent facts. This world is not all that there is. Isaiah Berlin defines the philosopher as "someone old who continues to think as a child."

In his classic treatise *The Child's Conception of the World*, Jean Piaget, the famed director of the Institut Rousseau and seminal theorist in child psychology, makes the point that the child's notion of reality is playful, exuberant, mythical, and mystical. When asked the very interesting adult question, "How does the sun move?" the child will give the fanciful answer, "God makes it move."[6] In contrast with our positivist worldview, the child has a "spirited" understanding. Perhaps this is what the Rabbi meant when he said, "Unless you become a child, you will not see the kingdom of heaven." The ethical import is that there may be a wisdom in naïveté and innocence. The great wisdom of literature of all ages written by the proverbial sage, who is usually a child though old in years, believes that there may be something beyond. Ethically speaking, to know both the beyond and within of life helps one choose wisely within the dialectic of aggression and acquiescence. Only awareness of God can properly guide us.

In hard clinical judgments the bearing of this insight about child perception is more complicated. We can impute to the child such innocence of worldview and faith instead of fear in the face of death and decide to let go without a struggle. One mother said she consented to a highly dangerous craniofacial surgery for her severely deformed child because she wanted him to die, go to heaven, and get his new body. Deranged theology can lead to deformed choice.

Another conflict of percepts that can occur and confound clinical decisions is found when parents and physicians share a strictly empiricist and materialist worldview which allows no transcendence. If life here is all there is, any and all treatments, no matter how desperate or caustic, should be tried. Sometimes such persistence is defended as benefiting future generations. But the tough ethical issue rises of using highly toxic treatments on this child, perhaps even hastening death, without much hope of cure or remission, in order to build a foundation of therapeutic knowledge to help other children in the future. In the ethical system we are espousing where themes of cohumanity, solidarity, fellow suffering, and trust in deliverance are dominant, such child sacrifice is possible, but only when checked by rigorous mechanisms of consent and victim advocacy.

Another reason to care actively and aggressively is the possibility of the unexpected, the miracle, even the spontaneous regression. In 1955 three surgeons wrote a remarkable case report. C. Everett Koop and William Kiesewetter joined with R. C. Horn to describe seven cases of cure and spontaneous regression of neuroblastoma among a total of forty-four children in which they only biopsied or partially removed the tumor.[7] Neuroblastoma is a very common tumor, especially in children under two years of age. Since surgeons Everson and Cole at the University of Illinois first reviewed spontaneous regression in various malignancies in 1966, numerous studies have shown a significant (2 percent) regression ratio and a dramatic responsiveness to treatment in the very young at an early stage of the disease.[8] The little we know of the rise and fall of malignancy suggests that there is miracle and grace in the continual devolution of tumor clones in our bodies, in the spontaneous cure, and in the blessed hard-won efforts of medical science in treatments cycles for the acute lymphocytic leukemia, Wilms' tumor, and other malignancies.

THEOLOGICAL ETHICS

Our discussion questions surrounding birth in its context of history, society, and the family can be explored from multiple perspectives, as we have seen. Theology, too, claims its due. Theology and its derived morality confirms us with a moral demand and a vision of possibility and prohibition that transports ethics from the time bound and narrow to a new level of insight.

Theology can be defined as the human mind's reception of the being and the word of God. Theology contributes to ethics as we receive the reality of God into the human soul at the site of the image of God and allow this communion to shape our own convictions (values) and our behaviors (virtues).

Throughout history, religion has demonstrated a strange paradox regarding the plight of children. On the one hand, religion has participated in the more general disregard and even dispatch of children by societies which were concerned mostly with their own survival. As we have discussed, many religions complied with practices of abortion and infanticide. When newborns were imperiled or abandoned, the church, through orphanages and hospices, was often involved in a ministry unto death. There is very little difference in the end result for the foundlings who came into the Montreal Hospital in the eighteenth century, where 92 percent died, and the Reich Children's Speciality Departments in the 1930s, where luminal sedation was given to unwanted children until they lapsed into comas and died.

Yet sometimes the church has been the most powerful source of new commitment to child life in its precious value and dignity. From this commitment have come the institutions of healing; the prohibitions of infanticide, homicide, and suicide; the ministries of orphan care and adoption; and of perhaps greatest impact, the teaching of communicant parents to love and honor their children.

Underneath this ambivalent moral posture is the paradoxical theology of child life and death. Christian thought celebrates life and health and vigorously opposes forces that would diminish or extinguish that gift. Christian faith also believes that we die unto the Lord. Death is not the absurd extinction of everything good and holy; it is rather deliverance from the power of sin and evil.

Theological ethics are shaped by this affirmation of life and the obligation to and for life. They are also counterchecked by the more ultimate devotion to God. In our creation we are both nature and spirit. In James Gustafson's words, our ethical obligations arise from our participation in the "patterns and processes of the interdependence of life," but fundamentally to those impulses "of what God is enabling and requiring us" to be and do within those life processes.[9]

Another general tension that is found in theological ethics relates to this primal responsibility to God and our world, the tension of obligation and forgiveness, law and grace, perfection and limitation. This dialectic calls us to strive but also to "let go." The immediate bearing of this bimodal conviction on decisions of impending death is obvious. A pediatric oncologist at M. D. Anderson once remarked that, when families with religious faith arrived on service, she breathed a sigh of relief. The hard experiences and decisions involving a dangerously ill child were so profound that such depth was required. Everything became much easier, she said—both the courage needed to intervene dramatically and the ultimate capacity to give up and take leave.

Again, related to this dichotomy is the fact that theological ethics complements natural reason. Ethics cannot be grounded solely on an ecological, biologic, philosophical, or theological basis. We need to see the complementarity of theological and natural perception, of revelation and reason. With reference to child life-and-death decisions, this means that risk-benefit and cost-benefit considerations are crucial but never sufficient. It also means that a perception about the will of God, though taken with utmost seriousness, need not become determinative.

Before we note how theological ethics transmutes through religious traditions, let us note a general secular development concerning serious child illness. In the old Roman Catholic cathedrals in South America, one can still find the attached orphanages with their "foundling wheels." These rotating cylinders built into the walls allowed a distressed mother or friend, without being seen, to place a baby on a round shelf, perhaps along with some clothes, money, and instructions on a lower shelf, and then turn the lazy-Susan-like tray around into the orphanage where the sick child or orphan would be taken and cared for. Like the partitioned confessional, this device acknowledged human frailty and inability to do what was required, in this case to care for seriously ill children. Not only orphanages and residences for the aged and infirm but also hospitals and clinics themselves are ways we acknowledge our insufficiency and moral incapacity to do, in the language of the *Prayerbook*, "what is meet and right." Such places of charity are antidotes to sin and sacraments of grace. Hospitality and hospitals embody by their very nature gestures of grace—they were not meant to generate wealth for stockholders but to care for others in our place. Through vicarious burden bearing we fill up the sufferings of the world (Col. 1:24).

A new piece of legislation has come before the U.S. Congress which attempts to embody this reciprocity with respect to one of the needs of severely ill and dying children. The Parental and Temporary Medical Leave Act of 1987, which came before the Senate Subcommittee on Children, Families, Drugs, and Alcoholism, requires employers with more than fifteen workers to provide up to eighteen weeks' leave with continued benefits to parents for the birth, adoption, or serious illness of a child. While we are not yet civilized enough to offer full pay for such leaves, as is the custom in some European countries, the bill will protect against unjust retaliation against working parents who leave work to come to the aid of a child. "We have a duty ... to support and protect our children," a guard at Cook County hospital commented. He had been suspended for a day and docked one day's pay when he left work to tend his seriously ill son.[10]

Theology is the human activity wherein we come to see and know God and in that encounter come to know our own exigency, our need and power (gift). That knowledge of self grounds ethics as it allows us to be given to one another in help. How does this transfiguration expressed in the theological ethics of religion find specific expression in the ethics of sick-child care? Religion is a developing radiance that begins with primitive wonder and proceeds through the great historic faiths, each enhancing and fulfilling the former.

Spirituality and religious morality as we know it takes its origins in Indo-European faith as expressed in the Indian continent. The theology of Hinduism revolves around three doctrines which in composite bear on our knowledge of God and our derivative ethical responsibility. *Karma* is the force of destiny by which our past and present actions continue to bear consequences into the future. *Samsara* is the Hindu doctrine of transfiguration, according to which, through rebirth of transmigration, the soul lives anew and lives on. *Moksa*, the doctrine of release or liberation, exposits the freedom in this faith even from the inevitability of *samsara* and *karma*. In this tradition the themes of the tragedy, transitoriness, and inevitable cycles of life stress resignation and submission to suffering. A certain apathy is found in the face of illness and suffering. Evil is absorbed in the deeper impersonal processes of the cosmos, and nobility of life is passion of spirit—warm, even sensuous, celebration of human vitalities and ultimately a release of the human spirit from striving.

A Hindu physician reflected on the theme of candor with patients as they were dying. "Every patient has the right," he argued (*right* having a very different meaning in Hindu theology than in Western jurisprudence), "to die under the illusion that he is getting better." A sick child in this medical philosophy is not extinguished in death; he or she merely passes through to another life. Whether or not illusion is fostered or at least not confronted in cases of serious illness or impending death, this belief system does affirm ongoing realities far greater than immediate suffering or death.

Through the mediating Egyptian spirituality, Judaism sustains the secular spirit from the precursor faith in the Asian and western

Asian subcontinents. But now God is not a vibrant and variegated pantheon of deities but a singular creative force of love and righteousness. The Jew extols the good life: health, well-being, delight, and moral justice. The Jewish command to enhance and protect life received from its giver and guardian is realistic about the human propensity to disregard, harm, and kill. To spill blood is to blaspheme, and for the physician to withhold services is to shed blood (Yoreh De^cah, 336:1). Evil is not impersonal but is a palpable human malevolence within each of our hearts. It also works out its malice in collectivities and nations. We must resolve to resist and counter such evil.

In Hebrew ethics children are honored and received as blessing. All resources of food and hygiene, health care and education, nurture, conversation, music, and the arts are presented for the flourishing of life. The commitment toward rich and full living disposes persons of this faith and ethic toward genetic screens to pick up defects and then abortion; for instance, there were more abortions than live births in Israel in 1982. The faith also inclines toward a philosophy of letting go and moving on to try again with imperiled newborns (e.g. Tay-Sachs). While official teaching, especially in orthodox and conservative circles, sustains the life-affirming and harm-protecting rhetoric, actual practice more often serves personal welfare and family viability. In the response to severe child illness and dying (e.g. to SIDS and malignancies), Jews, because of their faith and ethic, will be prominent in efforts to research and resolve the tragedies medically. They will philanthropically support institutes of exquisite care (such as children's hospitals). The psychology of perception will be more ameliorative than soteriological, seeking redemption from, rather than salvation through, suffering.

The Roman Catholic faith tradition expresses a more sacramental and salvific view of God and theological ethics. Judaism bequeaths the messianic impulse to the Christian tradition. The yearning for an anointed one who will come as deliverer and savior is shaped by the apocalyptic mood when history quakes with impending catastrophe. The God whom Israel meets when the soul and conscience had thus been made ready is a pathetic deity: a God who searches for the lost, cares for the wounded, avenges the poor and exploited, and suffers for and with those who suffer. The ethic that rises from this theology takes on new and different nuances and accents. A theology of incarnation invites the faithful to go down into the hard places of acute need, leaving the safe places of serenity and complacency and identifying with the afflicted. This condescension or incarnation is undertaken not so much to remove the pain but to participate with the victim(s) and be transformed by that suffering into redemption. Suffering, when received in cruciform faith, was liberating as it pointed to the beauty of resurrection and eternal bliss.

How might this new level of religious consciousness and its concommitant ethic respond to our tragic topic of moral perceptions about seriously ill and dying babies? Catholics found and sustain the Misericordia hospitals for severely sick, retarded, and handicapped children. When the pope climbed down from the stage of the Universal Amphitheater in Los Angeles to embrace Tony Melendez, the thalidomide victim who played his guitar with his feet, he praised Tony as "a sign of hope for the world." Melendez himself reflected Catholic piety when he responded, "I see my handicap as a state of blessing because I would not be doing what I am doing without it, which is my ministry in music."[11]

Islam also adds to the cumulative wisdom of theological ethics. This intense spirituality and ethic, born in the ancient Near East and now pervasive not only in Africa and Asia but throughout the Western world, can be seen as a puritan revulsion to Hellenic decadence. Ironically, it was apocalyptic Judaism, mediated through Abyssinian Christianity, that provided the crucible that refined Islam for its mission of destiny in world history. "Muhammed announced his divine call as *al Nabi al ummi*, the prophet to the nations ('barbarians'). He came in the authority of *Taurat* (Torah) and *Injil* (Gospel)."[12] Adherents of Islam believe that the divine nature shapes human nature through Allah's inexorable will, which is portrayed in the Koran as natural law. This prophetic theology and ethic believes that the human soul has direct access to the divine being and will. Medicine itself is both a divine gift and a human art. As such it is a ministry of strict theological observance. The great medieval scholars of Islamic medicine, which provided the bridge between the classical world of medical thought, practice, and theology and the modern traditions, spoke of "prophetic medicine." "Right intuition," which is the Islamic definition of ethical perception, is a mingled sense of the deep understanding of the human person as a mental-spiritual entity with the physical details filled in by scientific medicine and practical experience. Whether it be abortion, sexual therapy, care of children, human experimentation, or death care, this blended radiance of secular and sacred wisdom illumines each particular moral problem.

For the Koran the reality of God is morally confronted as our life in this world becomes the basis of judgment and resurrection. We must repent and renew life now in obedience and service. There is no allowance for deathbed repentance and forgiveness. The tradition is one of law and works-righteousness, all posited on a palpable inner sense of right and wrong.

> The entire Quran is directed towards inculcating in man a sense of "piety" or moral responsibility called *Taqwa* which literally means "to protect oneself" [against moral peril]. *Taqwa* is an instrument or an inner power which enables man to discriminate between right and wrong and to judge one's own actions. Ordinarily, men fail to judge their own actions properly because of deep layers of self-deception and self-righteousness such that even human conscience becomes colored by them.[13]

Conscience in the Islamic tradition is ordered by the severe justice of Allah. The moral demand always transcends our own tastes and preferences. It calls for austere obedience. There is not the tendency to domesticate conscience in Islam as there is in other world faiths. Moral will is heteronomous and theonomous. It comes from beyond. How does the faith perceive the child who is mortally ill? It searches for all of the benefits of medical science and pastoral care. It calls on all of the prophylaxes of diet, hygiene, and purification. Finally, it rests confident in the determinative will of Allah.

Like Islam, Protestant faith has been concerned with the distortions of conscience that riddle and confuse our subjective wills. Rather than perpetually seeking to justify ourselves by rationalizations or by strenuous worth-proving work (worship), the Protestant movement recovered the doctrine of justification by grace through faith. This doctrine, writes Carter Lindberg, has ramifications for medicine which include the following:

The divesting of "priestly" or sacred elements from medicine so that it may be rightly seen as penultimate.

The realization that life is not the highest good provides perspective on both health and illness.

The recognition of medicine's penultimacy may relieve both patient and therapist of false expectations.

The "alien righteousness" given persons by God stands against undue subjugation to technological manipulation or prolongation of life.

In the face of the ambiguities and failures (as well as successes) of life, the proclamation of the forgiveness of sins has particular relevance for the therapist as well as the patient.[14]

God is present to the soul as moral demand and as power equivalent to that demand. Nothing is called for that God is not able and willing to supply. The moral life is therefore one where perceptions are chastened so that we discern the moral call, and delusions of self-sufficiency are shattered so that grace can empower the good life.

As historians of Protestant culture point out, this tradition releases an enormous scientific and technological spirit. Human work in this impulse seeks to renew the world under the divine spirit. In Protestantism the Latin cross is emptied. The Lutheran cross is a powerful axis of shining steel, in vivid contrast to the bloody and burdened body-crucifix in the Mexican Catholic cathedral. Here serene strength displaces poignant pathos. Man has been reconciled to God. The distinctive value to proceed from this faith is "the eternal value of the individual and of his life" (Pannenberg). "God searches for every single individual like a sheepholder who goes after the one sheep that is lost until he finds it. It is like the poor woman who turns everything in her house upside down until she finds the lost coin. It is like the father who rejoices in the return of his lost son."[15]

The two ethical derivatives of this theology are the inestimable value of that single person, shielding that one from harm and proffering care and the future of the individual beyond death. When a child entrusted unto our care dies with SIDS or suffers with leukemia or neuroblastoma, we can be certain of two things: (1) we are called on to bring everything—our scientific, technological, and human power—to spare its life and save its future, and (2) paradoxically, or doxologically, we must say, nothing we do or that disease does can destroy that life.

Theological ethics are the necessary complement to the multi-faceted human morality we have described. They become especially pertinent when life's questions and crises are deep and hard. They bear a special relevance when we deal with children and when we deal with the finality of life. We know with children that we must hold on and provide but also sometimes let go. In his song cycle *Kindertotenlieder*, Gustav Mahler shares the outcry, the numbness, the trust:

In this weather, in this awful storm, I would never have let the
   children go out.
I was afraid they would die tomorrow; but there is nothing to
   do about that now. . . .
In this weather, in this storm, in this shower, they are resting,
Resting as if they were at home with mother. Frightened no
   more by storms,
Watched over by God's hand, they are resting as if they were at
   home with mother.

10 Eschatological Ethics of Safekeeping the Future:

CHILD NURTURE

Children begin by loving their parents; after a time they judge them; rarely, if ever, do they forgive them.

Oscar Wilde, *A Woman of No Importance*

Theology brings to our moral life an authority which supersedes the vitalistic reflections of ecology, biology, and the psychic and humanistic impulses inherent in philosophy, epistemology, history, and the law. Religion, jurisprudence, and literature all acknowledge the existence of a priority by which judgments are made; as Luther once declared, "my soul [conscience] is captive to the Word of God, God help me." In life we experience both appropriate and abusive authority. Luther's cry of conscience protests the wrongful authority of both church and state. Parents can also exert either edifying or detrimental stewardship. From the moment of a

167

baby's harsh expulsion into our world, imprinting begins, which im-
poses obligation on parents and elders. Even across species, newborns attach themselves to the nearest moving and nurturing
presence when separated from their mother. An orphaned duckling
will imprint to a human being or a dog. The process of instinctive
bonding to that one who will sustain you in dependence and then
release you in independence is a fundamental order of life. As the
epigraph from Oscar Wilde attests, it is a trust often violated by
both parents and children.

Our exploration now comes to its conclusion. We have examined the human drama of natality and nativity. We have seen human sexual and procreative power fashion much of the delight and
creative movement of civilization. We have also seen its dangers
and consequences. We have explored the moral issues of sexual being, being together, being with child, and being responsible for newborns and sick and dying children. Now we come to the issue of
offering children to this world and providing for them a world that
is safe and offers possibilities of fulfillment.

Two bishops of Rome reflect the manifold directions of ethics.
Eugene Kennedy's play *I Would Be Called John* reminded us of the
efforts of John XXIII to refresh, renew, and renovate the thought and
ethics of the church through the Second Vatican Council. Today another John, John Paul II, has met with American bishops to encourage them to be firm against dissent. He has reiterated his firm
message advocating justice for the poor, equality for minorities, and
mercy for the sick and oppressed. In many ways he is the child of
Vatican II. But in other ways his soul is fashioned, not in the warm
sun of a mountain village in northern Italy, but in the foreboding
gray atmosphere of communist Poland. He has called for the defense
of a view of God and the world and a way of life that he sees to be
threatened—from the East by godless state dehumanization and
from the West by a hedonistic materialism. His words now warn
against a world he sees as threatened by temptation and damnation—by divorce, adultery, abortion, homosexuality, greed, exploitation, technological degradation, and war. Ethics, as we saw from
these two bishops named John, like the broad system we have
sketched, can accent conservation, conformation, or liberation.

Our consideration of ethical theory moves now toward the pole
of liberation. Eschatology as a component of belief, and eschatological ethics, seeks the instruction of the new, that which has not yet
come to be but is coming, the future, the consummation. The
Greek word *eschatos* means "last" or "final." In theology eschatology is the science of the four last things: death, judgment, heaven,

and hell. In modern philosophy and historic parlance, the word has come to mean the consideration of that which is impending, the lure of futurity and possibility on contemporaneity and actuality. The *Oxford English Dictionary* has an interesting pejorative note at the end of its definition, one with which many modern skeptics would agree: "Eschatology, the science of the last things, is, as a science, one of the most baseless."

Eschatology is at once a very compelling and very dangerous dimension of ethics. On the one hand, it rescues us from an ethic that is purely nostalgic and conservative. By looking to the new and possible, an element of vitality and expectancy replaces the tedium of retrolineal and conventional stereotypes. But fanatics also use and abuse eschatological imagery: radio and TV evangelists saturate our airways and predict universal catastrophe. Those who pretend to know the future and control others by that knowledge are cautioned forever against that arrogance by the only one who ever lived for whom the future was complete ("Before Abraham was, I am" [John 8:58]). He said, "It is not for you to know the times or the seasons" (Acts 1:7). Robert Lifton, in his study of Nazi medical ideology, points to this eschatological perception, the transcendental state of consciousness which, as his subject shows, could be put to either healing or demonic effect. "The ultimate dimension addresses larger human involvements, the sense of being connected to those who have gone before and those who will follow our limited life span. We thus seek a sense of immortality . . . in what we look upon as eternal nature. The sense can be achieved by the experience of transcendence: of a special psychic state so intense that within it time and death disappear."[1] This individual and collective willingness of the Nazi time to lose self in some above or beyond was itself built upon an inner sense of loss, Lifton continues, an "ultimate breakdown in larger human connection."[2]

But eschatology does not only have to do with dread and doom. If one consults the literature of religious eschatology, political futurism, and science fiction, we also discover the benign and salutary side of the genre. We need to explore yet another moral crisis in our care for children: that of neglect, abuse, and abandonment of care for young children—the issue of forsaken future and violated hope.

THE CRISIS OF POSTNATAL AND INFANT MORTALITY

In 1987 the Food Research and Action Center released its 314-page report on hunger, which found that:

our progress in preventing infant deaths has come to a virtual
halt, despite the fact that advances in medical technology make
us capable of saving more and more very low birth-weight
babies ... from 1976 to 1981 infant mortality was reduced by an
average of 5% a year. In the 1981–1986 period that progress was
cut nearly in half. We believe that a large increase in hunger and
poverty in this period is a major cause of the slowdown. . . . The
major cities reported the highest infant mortality ... Washing-
ton, D.C. 21.2 infant deaths per 1000 live births. This was followed by Detroit (21), Atlanta (19.3), Newark (18.6), Cleveland
(16.9), Norfolk, VA (16.7), Baltimore (16.6), and Chicago (16.4).[3]

The ratio of children who die from preventable causes in the first
twelve months of life is 1 in 100. This ratio places the United States
well down on the list of nations in terms of infant mortality, beneath even some of the underdeveloped countries. The main cause
precipitating death is prenatal and postnatal malnourishment, causing low birthweight and rendering the baby vulnerable to all sorts of
infections and other diseases.

This report and others list the range of problems responsible for
this disgrace and the ameliorative efforts needed to resolve the
crisis, including the need to provide adequate nutrition to poor
mothers with children. In an editorial in the *New York Times*
a group of business leaders, educators, and economists issued a report which found the solution to the problem as one of simply doing something that works: concentrate on helping poor children in
their earliest months of life.[4] Table 1 lists programs that the *Times*
proposed.

Table 1
WIC: Food for Women, Infants, Children

Reduces infant mortality, increases birthweight. Participation: only a third of those eligible.	$1 spent on prenatal portion can save $3 in short-term hospital costs.

Prenatal Care

Increases birthweight and reduces premature births in mothers who otherwise forgo prenatal care in the first trimester.	$1 investment saves $3.38 in the cost of care for low birth-weight infants.

Medicaid

Reduces neonatal and infant illness and abnormalities through Early Periodic Screening, Diagnosis and Treatment Services. In 1986, 2.1 million were screened.	$1 spent on comprehensive prenatal care for Medicaid recipients saves $2 in first-year care.

Childhood immunization

Reduces rubella, mumps, measles, polio, diptheria, tetanus and pertussis. In 1983 more than 3.4 million children were immunized under the program.	$1 spent on childhood immunization saves $10 in later medical costs.

Preschool Education

Increases school success and employability and reduces dependence. Only 20 percent of those eligible participate in Head Start.	$1 spent on preschool education can save $4.75 in later social costs.

The moral crisis is in part political.

The administration folded maternal and child health programs into a block grant in 1982 and cut spending 18%. It cut spending for community health centers 13%. The WIC [Woman-Infant-Children] program provides diet supplements and checkups for poor pregnant and nursing women and their children—but it has only enough money to reach a third of those eligible. The administration now proposes more—a limit on Federal Medicaid grants to the states, and a cut that would drop a million participants from WIC.[5]

This indictment raises the critical question of parental obligations and state obligations to children. Is the administration responsible for this and all our problems? Some argue that the state takes on obligations for children only if it regulates procreation. In the case of Plato's *Republic*, where the state defines and delimits all procreation, it does indeed assume an obligation to protect and nurture those children. In the Western democracies, however, where the decision to have children is a private decision, the obligations of the state and state agencies and programs must rest on grounds other than taking care of what they brought into being. As table 3 shows,

a duty may arise from cost-benefit analysis and sheer self-interest—
the "pay now or pay later" doctrine. State programs may also be
seen as backup efforts or, to use the present metaphor, providing a
net through which no one will be allowed to fall. Proponents of this
view assume that, in procreation and childraising, parents ought to
be left alone, on their own and not interfered with either restric-
tively or remedially.

But when it comes to people needing help, this is an unrealistic
view of societal responsibility. We are inevitably members of communities and states. When human problems cannot be resolved by
familial, ecclesial, or private voluntary structures, they become
concerns of the society at large. To return to John Locke's doctrine
of parental responsibility or to create new legal fictions such as
grandparental obligation (grandmas are responsible for births to
their teenage daughters) is to deny the fact that the community—
city, state, nation—is the fundamental context of our living and
well-being, the absorber of life's hard knocks. When the body politic
is in a self-protecting and self-aggrandizing mood swing, as it now is
in the United States and the Western democracies, when the citizens say "I've had it" and refuse to pay any more taxes, we find it
hard to understand and accept these obligations, then elymosary
(almsgiving) and self-help structures have to be activated.

The main fallacy with the laissez-faire argument is that society
is involved in the social decisions that leave some people poor—
decisions about employment, education, welfare, and the living
deaths of premature babies. Four socioeconomic risk factors, factors
in part created by and remediable by the society, are involved:
the mother is less than twenty and single, did not graduate from
high school, and is receiving welfare support.[6] A good part of the
harm which exposes children to severe threat to life in the first year
has to do with our maturity, paternity, elymosary, and educabil-
ity values.

Before we turn to the global aspects of the crisis of presenting
children well into a world that will care, let us look at one other
aspect of the American ethos. It is now estimated that one half of
all children born in the United States are born into poverty. The
rate of children coming into families whose income is below the
poverty level is especially high among blacks and Hispanics. The
infant-mortality statistics among this community are shocking. But
even more alarming are the subtle and not-so-subtle deprivations
facing those who survive the first year of life. Minimal brain dys-
function, mild mental retardation, vitamin deficiencies and related

disorders, injured self-esteem, and debilitating fear and discourage-ment are but a few of the stigmata branded on children by a society that cannot muster the capacity to secure their lives.

Nor is all well with the wealthy. Equally painful are the middle-class pathologies which create the runaway and parental-rejection culture, depression, suicide, and the deadly combination of indul-gence and isolation where kids are given everything—except pre-cious time and involvement.

Though the national situation is calamitous, when we turn to the global perspective on providing a present and future world for children, we face nothing short of catastrophe. The 1986 *World Health Organization* statistics volume states the following:

> The first years of life are among the most hazardous in terms of survival chances. Poor sanitation, lack of safe water, overcrowd-ing, malnutrition and inadequate health care services often take a heavy toll on young lives. In several African countries, includ-ing Angola, Burkina Faso, Ethiopia, Gambia, Malawi, Mali, Mozambique, Sierra Leone and Somalia, as well as in Afghani-stan, more than one-quarter of newborns do not survive to their fifth birthday. Between 20 and 25 percent of infants die before age 5 in some countries of central and western Africa (Benin, Burundi, Central African Republic, Chad, Equatorial Guinea, Guinea-Bissau, Liberia, Mauritania, Senegal and Burundi), in Ye-men and Democratic Yemen, and in parts of south and east Asia (Bangladesh, Bhutan, Democratic Kampuchea, and Nepal). Throughout the remainder of Africa and Asia, the proportion of infants who fail to celebrate their fifth birthday typically varies between 10 and 20%. The exceptions include some Arab coun-tries (Jordan, Lebanon, the Syrian Arab Republic) as well as Burma, China, Mongolia, the Philippines, Sri Lanka and Thai-land, where between 5 and 10% do not survive to age 5. Infants in almost all countries of Latin America have at least a 90% chance of reaching their fifth birthday. This is not the case in Honduras, Guatemala, Nicaragua and Peru, where between 10 and 15% die before age 5, and in Bolivia and Haiti, where be-tween 15 and 20% do not survive. In a number of Latin Ameri-can countries, the proportion dying before age 5 is less than 5%, similar to the level prevailing in the developed world.[7]

In the most recent report of the *Epidemiological Bulletin* of the Pan American Health Organization, we see the sobering contrast of the rich and poor nations, a contrast covered over in routine inter-

American affairs such as the Pan American games in Indianapolis
(summer 1987) and political intrigues involving El Salvador and
Nicaragua. Tables 4–6 show the disparity of opportunity to survive
and thrive in the overdeveloped and developing worlds.

Three impressions arise from this data. In the first place, there
is a dramatic reduction in the devastation that life brings to children in the affluent parts of the world. We are beginning to approach that eschaton envisioned by a prophet called Isaiah over two
millennia ago.

> I will take delight in Jerusalem and rejoice in my people;
>   weeping and cries for help
>   shall never again be heard in her.
> There no child shall ever again die an infant,
>   no old man fail to live out his life;
>   every boy shall live his hundred years before he dies,
> . . . .
> My chosen shall enjoy the fruit of their labour.
> They shall not toil in vain or raise children for misfortune.
>   For they are the offspring of the blessed of the Lord
>   and their issue after them.
>   (Isa. 65:19–23 NEB)

Second, we have reason to hope for a future when infant death
will diminish even more among the earth's poor. Third, it appears
that development and affluence effects a trade-off of childhood mor-
bidities and mortalities. Consider seven vectors of mortality for
children under ten years of age: enteritis, influenza/pneumonia, avi-
taminosis, malignant neoplasms, homicide, accidents, and suicide.[8]
As a society becomes more affluent (developed, educated, wealthy,
etc.), the portion of the children who are "raised for misfortune"
diminishes, and the causes of infant and youth mortality change.
As a society improves its water supply, immunizations, nutritional
status, and health-care access, the former problems such as parasite
infestation diminish and the new ones like cancer and accidents
take their place. In a well society the major causes of child death
become homicides, accidents, and suicide.

What does this say about an eschatology of suffering? Some cyn-
ics or nihilists will use the arguments which invoke Sir William
Osler's description of pneumonia as "the old man's friend" and ask
whether the exchange of old diseases for new is progress. The reality
we face is one of more self-chosen rather than natural patterns of

Table 2

ARI-related deaths in children 0 to 4 years in 39 countries or areas reporting causes of deaths, according to level of infant mortality (in or around 1981).

Level of infant mortality (per 1,000 live birth)	Reporting countries/areas	Number of countries/ areas	Total popula- tion (millions)	Number of births per year (thousands)	Child population 0–4 years (millions)	Reported ARI-related deaths					
						Absolute figures			Rates per thousand		
						In infants	Children 1–4	Total	In infants	Children 1–4	Total
25 and less	**Northern America** United States, Canada	2	256.5	4,100	20.3	3,483	985	4,468	0.85	0.06	0.22
	Central America Costa Rica	1	2.4	74	0.3	352	97	449	4.59	0.39	1.43
	Asia a) Hong Kong, Japan, Singapore	3	126.0	1,638	9.0	2,003	1,097	3,100	1.2	0.20	0.34
	b) Israel, Kuwait	2	5.5	154	0.8	732	163	895	4.75	0.25	1.20
	Oceania Australia, New Zealand	2	18.3	296	1.5	291	88	379	1.00	0.07	0.30
	Europe	13	344.4	4,637	22.4	11,679	2,364	14,043	2.52	0.20	0.63
	Subtotal	23	753.1	10,899	54.3	18,540	4,794	23,334	1.70	0.11	0.43
26–50	**Americas**	4	46.1	1,183	4.9	8,804	2,118	10,922	7.44	0.6	2.23
	Asia	2	63.9	1,817	8.5	7,831	6,927	14,758	4.3	1.1	1.7
	Europe	3	55.2	945	4.6	15,722	2,972	18,694	16.6	0.8	4.1
	Subtotal	9	165.2	3,945	18.0	32,357	12,017	44,374	8.20	0.86	2.47
51 and over	**Americas**	6	46.9	1,800	7.6	22,873	20,071	42,944	12.7	3.46	5.65
	Asia	1	9.5	443	1.8	498	727	1,225	1.12	0.54	0.68
	Total	39	974.7	17,087	81.7	74,268	37,609	111,877			

Table 3
Annual number of deaths in children 0 to 4 years according to levels of infant mortality (global figures for 1981).

Level of infant mortality (per 1,000 live births)	Number of countries	Estimated total population (millions)	Estimated births per year (millions)	Estimated child population 1–4 years (millions)	Estimated global number of deaths (millions)	
					In infants	In children 1–4 years
25 and less	51	1,127	16.0	67.5	0.3	0.10
26–50	27	1,451	31.3	122.0	1.3	0.35
51–75	9	190	6.5	21.7	0.4	0.15
76–100	20	470	17.4	55.8	1.6	0.60
101–125	18	1,110	41.2	120.0	4.6	2.40
126 and over	25	252	11.6	33.0	1.8	1.00
Total	150	4,600	124.0	420.0	10.0	4.60

Table 4
Five leading causes of death with rates per 100,000 in children 1–4 years, in countries with highest rates in this age group, 1978.

Country	Order				
	1st	2nd	3rd	4th	5th
Guatemala	Enteritis 408.6	Influenza Pneumonia 220.5	Measles 121.2	Whooping cough 39.1	Avitaminosis 44.1
Ecuador	Enteritis 227.5	Bronchitis 91.2	Influenza Pneumonia 89.9	Avitaminosis 38.3	Accidents 37.3
Honduras	Enteritis 92.8	Measles 41.6	Influenza Pneumonia 34.8	Bacillary dysentery 18.7	Bronchitis 14.6
Peru	Enteritis 134.2	Influenza Pneumonia 104.2	Bronchitis 34.3	Measles 32.1	Avitaminosis 25.3
Paraguay	Enteritis 198.7	Influenza Pneumonia 65.2	Accidents 27.2	Avitaminosis 20.1	Bronchitis 11.6

morbidity and mortality, heightened excruciation in some ways (is cancer preferable to bronchial pneumonia?), more exquisite forms of suffering (neurological, emotive, psychic), and greater challenge for sympathetic consolation. As civilization advances, we will be vexed more and more about the meaning of suffering. As various etiologies come to light, we will come to know both the inevitability of disease and death and our own complicity in its genesis. We will be able to remedy some sources of disease and death only by substituting others. Indeed, it is likely as we reach the end of this millennium that the dominant diseases in the Western world will be AIDS and Alzheimer's. In times like these, a contemplation of final purposes and meanings will then become an irrepressible quest. As we become more "godlike," we will possess more decisive power over birth and death.

This realization of newfound power and responsibility encourages world bodies like the United Nations and the World Health Organization to bring the nightmare of infant mortality and child loss under the eschatological judgment of a blissful vision such as that expressed in the *United Nations' Declaration of the Rights of the Child* (1959).

Principle 2—The child shall enjoy special protection, and shall be given opportunities and facilities, by law and by other means, to enable him to develop physically, mentally, morally, spiritually, and socially in a healthy and normal manner and in conditions of freedom and dignity.

Principle 4—The child shall enjoy the benefits of social security. He shall be entitled to grow and develop in health; to this end special care and protection shall be provided both to him and his mother, including adequate prenatal and postnatal care. The child shall have the right to adequate nutrition, housing, recreation, and medical services.

Principle 6—The child shall ... wherever possible ... grow up in an atmosphere of affection and of moral and material security. Society and the public authorities shall have the duty to extend particular care to children without a family and to those without adequate means of support. Payment of state and other assistance toward the maintenance of children of large families is desirable.[9]

The child, by virtue of its being brought into the world or, in Heidegger's phrase, having been cast unwillingly into existence, is entitled to a safe and provident home. Some will say that this child, or this many children, ought not to have been brought into the world. Yet these children are here with us. In the miracle of divine allowance, they have been granted entry into our world. They are now our trust. Confusing the issue of contraception or even abortion with this question, condoning neglect by saying that such children ought not to have been born, is absolutely unconscionable. In our ethical view life emerges from the mystery of origination and moves toward the mystery of destination. Our ethical responsibility as a human community is to provide safe passage.

By both omission and commission child abuse in our national and global culture is a moral scandal. Ethics involves concerns about who we actually are and what actual harm is being done. It also involves the parents and adults that we should or could be—an eschatological ingredient of ethics. In their important collection of essays on the ethics of child care, Onora O'Neill and William Ruddick speak of this dual nature of responsibility in the area of child abuse.

> The most publicized cases of child abuse and neglect are lurid tales of sadism and torture. But these are not the cases likely to help us think carefully about abuse and neglect. No one doubts the need for some form of state intervention to protect children from parents (or others) who starve or batter them. Doubts arise when one considers homes which are less dramatically deficient—for example, homes which are filthy or unstimulating, or where a parent has psychiatric or other health problems or perhaps is criminal or promiscuous.[10]

None of us is in fact what we ought to be or could be. We all bear lethal and fatal flaws in our personality and in our actions. Ethics, in one sense, is bringing our lives into sympathy and complementarity so as to soften one another's rough edges, make up for one another's deficiencies, blunt each other's potential malice, and together absorb suffering and meet need. The "new being" of religious teaching is the individual and collective entity which, through helping response to need, transfigures suffering and death into new life.

Something inherently futuristic or eschatological is involved when we speak about parents, elders, and children. The moral genius of this association involves living together toward something new. As William Ruddick points out, the dominant parenting metaphors of "producers" and "guardians" need to be enriched by metaphors which convey the themes of opportunity, freedom, and possibility. He proposes that we think of our generational privilege in terms of a "prospect provision principle."[11] When we consider this image of opening life options, of generating in our children powers of competence, discernment, and consideration, we move into what can best be called eschatological ethics.

ESCHATOLOGICAL ETHICS

Eschatological ethics is the counterpart of the apocalyptic. The eschatological is justice (judgment) bearing crisis in time and history as apocalyptic is justice bearing crisis in space and nature. When our moral concern with children turns to preparing a future, we are involved in moral expression across time and history.

When we turn to the theme of eschatology, we are faced with some of the same fantastic and otherworldly images that we found when we spoke of apocalyptic. Though all cultures from the primitive communities down to communist bureaucracies express some form of eschatology (images of judgment, future, hope), the ideas lack credibility today for those who seek a language of universal reason and science. Can we show that eschatological considerations are essential to ethics (Pannenberg)? This can be accomplished only if we can establish that the eschaton is a valid aspect of reality and if eschatological perception is an integral component of moral consciousness—the culminating constituent of ethics.

The first distinction that must be drawn is that found between secular and spiritual eschatology. Commenting on Pope John Paul's 1987 visit to the United States, philosopher Michael Novak noted that the pope had chosen as his theme "the primacy of the Spirit," that is, the power of the human spirit in history.[12] Both secular and sacred eschatology believe in the power of the human spirit to transform history. For the secularist, eschatology has to do with free human decisions which shape the future. Spiritual eschatologies have to do with the reality of God's impinging from the future onto the present. Karl Marx took Hegel's eschatology, which was a blending of Greek idealism and biblical expectancy, and fashioned a materialistic, this-worldly eschatology. A closer view shows that Marx was part of a more general trend in the nineteenth century which favored the religious tradition of realized eschatology as opposed to futuristic eschatology (Schweitzer). Realized eschatology emphasized the element of human work and social transformation in bringing into being the kingdom of God here and now. One can also make distinctions among individual, national, and universal futures and finalities.

The source of eschatological understanding in Western culture is the Greek view of the good as articulated by Socrates and the Hebrew-Christian view of God as the good and the future, comingled in the reality called "the kingdom." In the Socratic doctrine of the good we find the legacy of ancient Hellenic mystery faiths joined with the high reaches of rational philosophy in the fifth century B.C. The good is what people know they lack and therefore search after. In some sense, the good marked the discrepancy between value and being. Plato spoke of the good as "beyond being." The Greek understanding of "the good" was not some mysterious, elusive quality. Rather, it was simply the quality that reified people's desires about what was good for them. Philosophers like Kant criticized classic philosophy on the ground that it was a superficial "eudaimonism," a desire for happiness. But satisfaction is both elusive and inadequate to the moral excellence of persons. Aristotle transformed Greek thought and rendered the quest for and achievement of virtue as the essence of happiness. In the New Testament Scriptures, this Socratic and Aristotelian concept died, as the evangelist Matthew spoke of simple and radical righteousness as the essence of blessedness (Matthew 5–7).

Also behind this radical text, which has been called "the charter of human happiness," is the Judaic eschatology. Scholars find two sources of Hebrew teaching: preexilic and postexilic. In the prophets of the eighth century, the people of Israel receive teaching about God and his demand for justice and righteousness and the establishment of his authority and dominion. Amos, Hosea, and Isaiah speak of God's plan of salvation for the people—a coming salvation that will be ushered in by a time of judgment. In the post-exilic prophets (Deutero-Isaiah, Zechariah), the kingdom is given universal magnitude and salvific (healing) character as it establishes peace in the midst of darkness and danger. "Behold my servant, whom I uphold, my chosen, in whom my soul delights; I have put my Spirit upon him, he will bring forth justice to the nations . . . to open the eyes that are blind, to [release] the prisoners" (Isa. 42:1, 7 RSV).

The New Testament throughout is an eschatological and apocalyptic literature. It expects the imminent end of the world, as this is implied as the kingdom of God ruptures into our world and experience. The preaching, teaching, healing, and miracle working of Jesus is understood by the primitive Christian community as the inauguration of the messianic kingdom and the onset of end time. The great architect of Christian theology after Paul the apostle is Augustine. In the fourth century A.D., as the Goths, Visigoths, and Vandals were sweeping across western Europe, Augustine formulated the theology of time and history which became the normative eschatology for Christian civilization. For Augustine, the end of life, the summum bonum, is no longer happiness but God. Put another way, ethics and philosophy now discover true happiness in life with God. In fact, the fundamental intellectual and spiritual discovery that he makes is that God *is* the good. No longer is the good separate from people and God. The good is no longer happiness; it is the human being living for God. In striving toward God, one lives into the future, into judgment. "The condition for the hope of future happiness is commitment to God. When this order is reversed and one chooses his own happiness instead of God as the goal of existence we have, according to Augustine, the precise definition of sin. Thus the structure of the ethical quest as described by Aristotle is the description of man's sinfulness.... The good is to be seen as the future, yet to be fulfilled."[13]

The moral life is life proceeding onward toward the mark. Sin is misdirection, moving off target, falling away. Eschatology now becomes the essence of ethics. God's impending judgment becomes a judgment on himself. Where his life is manifest, we find the good. Where God is not honored as present, evil and sin prevail. God is human good, and human good is God. When this conjunction is understood, it is no longer possible to affirm a dualism or pessimism about this world. In the eschaton, which is the good as it breaks back toward us from the future, God is all in all (Col. 3:11). Otherworldly eschatology leads to disparagement and disregard for his world. The original Christian eschatology, by contrast, is directed into this world toward its transformation. Here we see the connection of eschatology with ethics and with the commitment to a world made safe and fulfilling for children.

The two significant moral ideas that derive from eschatology are the dominion of God and the reality of penultimate and ultimate judgment. Though these ideas have faded from modern consciousness, they still bear moral currency. The relevance of the reign or dominion of God over world structures and systems and over human life is obviously a preeminent ethical factor if the presuppositions of the affirmation are granted. Such theocratic assumptions cannot automatically be applied, especially in modern secular and pluralistic states. But the kingdom of God as an ethical criterion does deserve more serious attention than is our custom in according it "spiritual" significance alone. When Jesus said, "The kingdom is within you," he indeed meant to affirm the necessity of interior and existential fealty in our response to "kingdom come." It is also certain that these words were not intended to relegate our reception and creation of God's kingdom to pious aspects of the inner life and life after death.

Theology and theological ethics in recent years have become strongly eschatological. As we become aware of our power over the future and more certain of our obligations to history and to those who will follow after us, we also become aware that our religious and moral traditions, at least in the Abrahamic faiths (Judaism, Christianity, Islam), disclose to us a God who acts with moral effect in history. The theology of hope and futurity and historical and eschatological ethics gained expression in the 1960s by Catholics such as Karl Rahner and Johannes Metz and Protestants like Jürgen Moltmann and Wolfhart Pannenberg. In the late 1970s and early 1980s, the unbending pathos of human suffering cast another light on the liberating hope of that earlier theology and ethic. Eschatological theology generated liberation theology. The desperate plight of persons in Africa, Asia, and Central America, the desperation of the past even in the bosom of the highly developed and affluent societies, the failure of society to grant meaningful equality and opportunity for women, the agony of abortion and AIDS, and the sad underside of modern affluence and opulence all brought a plaintive note of suffering to our eschatology. In the theology of Johannes Metz, for example, that which makes us human, our connection with the background and the future of the race, is participation in human suffering. What he calls the "dangerous memory of Jesus," the receipt into our moral consciousness of the eschatology of the Last Supper, binds us in memory and hope to the plight of the oppressed, the wounded, and the sinner—the world for whom Christ would die. If the coming kingdom is envisioned in evolutionary terms and we hope for the gradual realization of a new and better world, a constructive ethic emerges to build that future. But if the kingdom is viewed as discontinuous with the present and the transcendent, any moral gestures will be symbolic rather than systemic. In either case the divine dominion becomes both the substance and the authority of ethics.[14]

A second theme of eschatological ethics is the reality of judgment. The fundamental ground of ethics across the ages has been the hope of reward and salvation and the fear of punishment and damnation. Today the structure of heaven and hell, certainly as features of the external physical landscape and as specific places above and under the earth, has broken down. Even the reality of a good and evil as structures of moral consciousness has waned. But the idea that peace, good conscience, and happiness is the reward of righteousness, and conversely that discontent, guilt, and sadness will be the aftermath of malevolent wrongs still carries an empirical currency.

In the same way we continue to believe that, in some ultimate sense, immortality supplies justification for the good life. The doctrine of grace and judgment, reward and punishment, heaven and hell, had to be cleansed from its immoral aspect, whereby one would do good not out of genuine kindness or justice but to manipulate a reward. In the same way, to act solely out of fear of punishment is not morally worthy. Only a realized or contemporaneous eschatology can undergird moral excellence. In this case one acts out of compassion for another without lust for reward or fear of punishment, absorbing evil and releasing good out into the human cosmos, the here-and-now world, which is the true arena of divine redemption.

When eschatology is ethically conceived in this way, we avoid the two dangers of taking justice into our own hands because the gods and the state have failed or, conversely, abandoning justice to some extrinsic or posttemporal retribution. It is our task in this life and this world to do justice and to love mercy (Micah). In her book *Wild Justice*, Susan Jacoby claims that vengeance becomes necessary when faith in the divine righteousness and the human structures of justice have failed. In a moving editorial, Otto Friedrich writes of the futile hunt for Josef Mengele with the perverse benediction "Non requiescat in pace." The need for justice, Friedrich states "lies at the heart of tragedy." As Orestes avenged the murder of Agamemnon and Hamlet postponed his own revenge on Claudius until the usurper could be killed while sinning, then "his soul might lie as damn'd as hell whereto it goes," Friedrich continues:

> The cruelest imagined torments of hell once seemed not only very real but a perfectly legitimate form of punishment, since God himself had permitted and even approved the eternal fires. And with what a hunger for retribution did Dante identify each king or warrior he reported seeing in the Inferno, buried up to the eyes in rivers of blood. With what zeal did Bosch and Bruegel similarly portray malefactors being torn at by giant birds or

skeletons. Yet the avenger himself was traditionally punished too. Orestes goes mad; Hamlet dies of poison; Captain Ahab ends in a tangle of rope dragged by Moby Dick. Revenge is both necessary and forbidden. In the case of Mengele, the social contract that promises justice did seem to have failed.[15]

Thomas Jefferson, though a son of the Enlightenment, retained some vestige of the classical and biblical theology. He wrote, "I fear for our nation when I ponder the truth that God is just. His justice cannot sleep forever."[16] Elie Wiesel, Anne Frank, and the other child-victims of the Holocaust dreamed of the same ultimate vindication out of their indomitable spirit of justice and right. The eclipse, silence, or sleep of God must not be construed (as did Nietzsche) as the death of God but as the divine accession to our freedom and responsibility. In the suppression of tyranny, the exposure of falsehood, the rescue and safeguard of victimized innocents, and the condemnation of contemptuous disregard for those dependent on us, we must act as if we were on our own but confident that divine righteousness will ultimately prevail.

We are either the advocates or the abusers of children. Apathetic withdrawal or laissez-faire resignation to supposedly benevolent or malevolent inevitability is irresponsible. It is our responsibility to fashion for them that good and safe world of our noblest hope.

Synthesis

I have hoped to offer a fresh, deep, and incisive conceptual structure for bioethics, one which would illumine certain clinical and policy questions. That contemporary bioethics theory is not adequate to the issues at hand is now widely acknowledged. While it is clear that the times call for a richer, more multifaceted ethical theory to address adequately the questions of the day, the rush of issues has forced us to call on the well-worn principles of analytic philosophy: autonomy, beneficence, and justice. Regrettably these principles are usually invoked, stripped even of their own historic and normative depth and correlated with the perennial schools of morality: utilitarianism, deontology, and natural law.[1] A breakthrough in ethical theory has been foreshadowed for years by many developments, including the amplification of the analytic perspective in philosophy with the revival of political and virtue theory,[2] the emergence of biologic theory,[3] and the new power of theological theory.[4]

As I hope to have shown in this study, a more sensitive understanding of patient suffering and physician caring has arisen with the broader understanding of the pathos of history and metaphysics. The term *ethics* signifies the discernment of good and evil in the universe. It has to do with responsibility in the interactions between and among people. The heart of medical ethics, therefore, lies in the redemptive meeting of selves at the axis point of suffering and salvation which sickness creates. The breakthrough notion of ethics we have proposed has proven to be, we trust, more responsive to the sociohistorical and therapeutic consciousness of our time.

A medical ethics for our time must be true to the reality it purports to comprehend. This means that it must respond to both the agonal expression of human need and the ameliorative nature of medical care. Human ethics are interrelational. They refer to being, value, and deeds, person to person. Obligation or moral action may

185

be defined as need which calls for help. The essence of ethics is responsibility, responsiveness, or even *Verantwortlichkeit* (intense answerability). Simone Weil has written, "The world needs saints who have genius, just as a plague-stricken town needs doctors. Where there is a need, there is an obligation."[5] Medicine, as the French origins of the word suggest, involves science, technique, and healing. The ethical motive of the art and the act of medicine is therefore shaped by that which it can do and that which it is meant to be.

SUFFERING SORGEN: A LEITMOTIF FOR ETHICS

If ethics has to do with the dealings between persons and is therefore by its very nature transactional, then the moral essence of medicine has to do with the genius of that poignant meeting of a call of need from a sufferer with one competent to help and willing to care. Medical ethics, then, represents a resonance of patient confession with physician and nurse profession. This juncture of patient pain and clinician care, when characterized by abiding, altruistic, and agapic concern, mimics a fundamental normative (historical, natural, and transcendental) quality of reality itself. The German verg *sorgen* and the noun *Sorger,* which call to mind the primitive nurse or healer, are words which convey constancy graced with power, a kind of attendance which sacramentally participates in the deeper mystery of being where brokenness yields to wholeness and death is transformed into life.

To fathom the metaethical context of meaning that has been proposed here as the foundation of ethics, we first need to affirm a series of normative propositions. These may be stated in the following order:

1. Crucifixion, or moral crisis involving the sacrifice of the good momentarily to evil so that good may eventually prevail, occurs when the spiritual realm meets the physical and future succeeds past.
2. Holocaust, a dimension of cruciform reality, is a pervasive pattern in history.
3. Suffering must therefore be at the center of any normative understanding of the meaning of human existence.
4. Suffering, death, and transfiguration form the normative pattern of reality, which is noetically superimposed on actual reality.

5. Suffering patience, redemptive amelioration, and sympathetic participation are morally fitting responses to this supernal reality.

What do these metaphysical thoughts have to do with the ethics of natality? Simply this: the moral questions that have confronted us in the sphere of perinatality, issues such as human sexuality, birth, and child life, are events in space, time, and eternity. Since ethics seeks to discern the inner direction and normative quality of space, time, and eternity and to find moral direction not only from the ideal but also of the accessible reality, we seek to discern those parameters of what we know in order to make right choices. Reality as we know it presents itself in the dimensions of space, time, and eternity. Prescriptive reality emerges from this descriptive reality. We therefore have taken these three dimensions and have sought the natural, temporal, and supernal renditions of the normative leitmotif we have claimed to be definitive for ethics. We have unfolded this ethical structure in the ten dimensions of ethics that we have touched on in the clinical chapters. These dimensions express the tripod foundation (*physis, tempus, aeternitas*) which we contend is the necessary conceptual basis for ethics. Let us now in summary revisit these threads of moral fabric and weave them, then, in conclusion into our garment of one piece, a shalom quilt.

REQUIREMENTS OF A NEW ETHIC

There are more things in heaven and earth, Horatio, than are dreamt of in your philosophy.

Shakespeare, *Hamlet*

A broad and nuanced ethical approach needs to be developed if we are to be able to inform personal and public decision making for the perinatal crises that await us in the waning years of this millennium. The required revision in our conceptual structure of ethics has been explored throughout this volume. In each chapter we explored one feature of the theory in conjunction with a specific problem area. The thesis developed can be expressed as follows: To be ethical, a personal or policy decision should be appropriately ecological, apocalyptic, biologic, psychic, philosophical, epistemic, historical, legalistic, theological, and eschatological. These dimensions of reality communicate with the moral soul through the following capacities: mimetic, threnodic, animistic, psychological, rationalistic, phronetic, anamnetic, political, pietistic, and elpistic.

DIMENSIONS OF ETHICS

The cosmic, *ecological*, or environmental aspect of ethics is the ground level of morality. "Going with" and not "going against" nature is perhaps the most primal moral imperative. The world is the setting of our life. We live in a life-world where all interactions impact the whole. We live in a natural environment where cycles of replenishment must be honored lest overconsumption despoil and exhaust the commons. The cosmos displays to us not only vast indifference but also splendidly harmonious patterns of cause and effect, providence, restoration, venture, and consolidation. The display in human conscience provides a bedrock for ethics.

The *apocalyptic* dimension may sound strange and out of place. Yet it always has been and retains yet today a central place in the geography of ethics. Apocalypse is crisis or trauma or possibility within nature itself. The great apocalyptic stories which appear in all cultures, especially in the Hebraic, Greek, and primitive Christian literatures, speak of cataclysm, end time, ultimate judgment, and the final rupture of the heavens and earth. If creation and cosmos emit signals of acceptance, boundaries, and serene accommodation and this becomes the character of ecological ethics, apocalypse conveys expectancy, judgment, and disruption. Judgment and prolepsis—what should have been and what could be—are further bases for ethics.

The *biologic* vector of morality has recently come under careful study and has yielded some remarkable insights into human ethics. Decisions to allow defective newborns to die recall primitive human infanticide and animal abandonment. Impulses to protect and nurture offspring, even at great sacrifice, have similar roots in our biologic substance. Impulses of sexual intimacy and procreation arise from such deep genetic and instinctive springs of our behavior that we cannot retrieve their origins.

A mother was unwilling to accept the fact that her baby was not going to survive. She continued to insist on artificial life supports long beyond any hope her child might recover. Finally she decided to give the baby a period of time to see if it would show any natural impulse to recover. After this failed, she was willing to let the baby go. This instinct, like the trial or ordeal of suspect offspring among animals, where the mother sets the little one out on its own for a test of strength before she reestablishes nurture, was a fitting response, a biologic impulse well heeded.

Rising within the biologic dimension and extending to new levels is the *psychic* dimension. Here we begin to see what makes us free and moral beings. Impulses rooted in our biologic being are refined and sublimated into emotions that are a major force in stimulating behavior. Think of the importance for the moral life of love and hate, guilt, shame, joy, and hope. The pain/pleasure axis, while originating in the biologic stratum of our existence, is most fully realized in the psychological. The affirmation that something is right or wrong because it feels good or it hurts has come under strong attack in modern ethics. The argument that I like or dislike a particular action or outcome and therefore it is right or wrong does not carry much weight on the Pediatric Bioethics Committee or in the court of law. However, the psychological realm does press toward the point where we can ascertain as valid or invalid a given choice because determinations can be made regarding knowledge and intent of action. Psychology also has the ability to discriminate (as Erik Erikson does, for example) between the healthy or unhealthy (stagnating) choice or inclination.

The human mind also is the seat of the *philosophical* and *epistemic* capacities for ethical judgment. In one sense, all ethics proceed through the channels of philosophy or political philosophy. In classical times, philosophy was a wisdom that embraced all sources of human insight. Natural philosophy was the home of the sciences; moral and political philosophy subsumed a range of other disciplines offering insight into truth. Today, however, philosophy has assumed a more modest role, more critical and supportive of other modes of insight and less willing to be the vehicle of *sophia* than it was in other intellectual eras.

In this book we have asked philosophy to assume tasks of definitional precision and analytic coherence but also those of theoretical and practical wisdom. The Greeks used several different words whose meanings we draw together in our concept. *Epistēmē, doxa, sophia,* and *phronēsis,* among others, refer to those capacities of calculation, extrapolation, judgment, and common sense that together constitute our moral psychology. The bicameral mind helps us to think in the two modes critical to moral reflection. There is the realm of logic, causality, consistency, coherence, and sequence. Here the traditional powers of moral reasoning are needed. What are the outcomes to be expected from certain actions? Then there is the more subtle task of moral reasoning: to embrace paradox, the un-known, and mystery. How do these elusive realities contribute to moral choice?

For the general moral issue of dealing with concurrent knowl-edge and ignorance, we have called on quantitative intelligence, utility reasoning, and moral calculation. We will call this skill epistemic moral intelligence. The more general humanistic tradi-tion of philosophy, the ethics of human freedom in the Kantian mode, the ethics of the great bioethical principles—autonomy, be-neficence, and justice—take us into the realm of sophia (wisdom). This is the more fundamental meaning of philosophy.

For the Greeks the word anamnēsis referred to the liberating in-sight of recollection or remembrance. This word speaks of the ethi-cal value of the historical perspective. Memory is a crucial component of the ethical structure of our consciousness. If cosmic and apocalyptic perspectives ask, Where do we come from? and bi-ologic, psychic, philosophical, and epistemic perspectives ask, Who are we? the historical perspective asks, Where have we been? The three final perspectives to follow—political, theological, and escha-tological—will find the good in part addressed by the questions, Who are we? Who might we be? and Where are we going?

We are also a part of a social organism. We are members of the polis. We are inevitably social and political creatures, and this gives rise to another component of the moral sense. We next considered the legalistic dimension of ethics. Conscience (suneidēsis) and re-sponsibility, by their very definition, involve reciprocity and com-munity. Freud spoke of the sway that a primordial historical collective consciousness still had on our believing and valuing self. Rousseau and the Romanticists projected back into the early times of human history structures of covenant and social contract that grew out of primal senses of community obligations. Moral cogni-zance of others and of their expectations, taboos, rules, and sanc-tions all structure what we call conscience. The virtues of solidarity, continuity, and altruism as well as the vices of conven-tionalism, conformity, and legalism arise from this part of the moral soul. At this level we considered the necessary influence of law, politics, economics, and social values on our ethics.

The theological dimension of ethics was one of the most diffi-cult to justify and clarify. Critical philosophers argue that we can-not rationally verify values that are based on a divine word or will. They further claim that religiously grounded ethics are hopelessly pluralistic, even contradictory. We are therefore left with a dilemma.

While we must appeal to transcendence because of the limits of natural reason and the contingency of "extremis" decisions, in theological ethics we cannot arrive at certainty or consensus. In this book we have explored a different approach to theological ethics and religious traditions. On the basis of a sequential and developmental interpretation of the history of religions, we have argued for a universal ethic that is more than a synergistic or "least common denominator" position. The following proposal about how to read religious history is not meant to be some profound revision of *Religionswissenschaft*; it is simply a common-sense look at the religio-moral experience of humankind, extracting and distilling what seems to be not only a universal wisdom but also a sense of where we have arrived in the believing history of human communities.

We have proposed the following sequence of events in religious history which further influences not only parochial but universal ethics:

simple primitive mystic superstition emergent whenever enclaves of people appeared;

the coalescence of a conquering Indo-European movement;

the ecstatic yet sensuous spirituality of Hinduism;

the emergence of high religion in Egypt, Israel, and western Orient;

the spontaneous eruption of the great eighth-century prophetisms;

the serene wisdom of the Greek *oikoumenē* into which Christianity appeared, bearing universal power into Judaism;

the insertion of Islam to amplify Abrahamic faith in the Arabic world, passed over by Christianity in its rapid gravitation to the Occident;

the resurgence of Eastern Christianity;

the Reformation within the Western church, detailing fine points of belief and ethics in a magnificent spray of emphatic visions;

the nineteenth-century sects, responding to secular tendencies and sounding missing notes in the grand symphony;

now all branches of faith, Eastern and Western, oscillating into fundamentalist and modernist tones to satisfy the enormous thirst of the twentieth century for both pure faith and radical freedom.

Through a certain naive uncomplicated concave lens, one can look at the history of religion in this way.

What does this story line of faith mean for ethics? The variety of world faiths not only expresses an ethnic, racial, and cultural diversity and reflects the rich complication and mystery of the very being of God, it also recognizes the profundity of the moral imperative. Intensified and diversified faith signals the wonder and terror of the mystery of divine will in life and death and in the life course of persons and peoples. Faith, in one sense, is the working out of moral clarification.

Religion is a universal phenomenon. Not only is it evident that humans are by nature *Homo religiosus,* but there is also a universal substance to theological truth. Although the cultured despisers always try to repudiate faith on the basis of accused subjectivity and relativity, in fact theology has made a truth claim on all persons regardless of the particular beliefs to which people adhere. Much of religious diversity is trivia, trappings and tangential accents of belief and value which all persons of faith acknowledge to be insignificant when viewed in the light of major issues. Examples of universal convictions that all faiths would affirm include:

the existence and presence of God;

the moral imperative;

the human soul as receptor of this imperative and embodiment of the image of God;

the reality of immanent and impending justice;

the fact of human malevolence and apathy.

To round out the full orb of ethics, we open the human spirit to the *eschatological* realm. Here, through the faculty of hope (*elpsis*), we touch and are touched by that which is not yet but is coming to be. Here we experience new quality of being as we live not only bound to past and present but open to what could and might be. In Ernst Bloch's powerful phrase, we become creatures of *Ontologie des noch nicht Seins* (ontology of being that is not yet). In the human spirit *elpsis* is always found in delicate interaction with *phobos* (fear). We can project futures that are ameliorative and redemptive, worth striving for or waiting for. We can also construct imaginary worlds or conditions which can drain the verve of life and through disappointment bring the obverse of hope (*spes, speris*), despair.

In some sense all ethics culminates on the eschatological plane. Every decision is de novo; it has never happened before. In one sense decisions are forces that change the future. Our decisional life is that which creates the new. Eschatology has this generic sense and at that level anchors the ethical powers of prediction, feedback reading, and consequence mapping. In another sense eschatology refers to "last things." In strains similar to our discussion of apocalyptic, we ponder here final outcomes, the denouement of nature and history as space and time collapse back into eternity. Both senses of eschatology are morally instructive. Feedback or anticipation of effects of actions is an essential ingredient of the utility requirement of ethics. The fact that all things pass away enforces the sense of transiency, which in life-and-death questions is basic to wisdom.

SUMMARY

We have introduced what we contend are the vital dimensions of ethics, factors which should be consulted in every moral decision. We need today Benedictine-like disciplines of contemplation and action that will make such consideration of changing impulses instinctive and second nature. We now conclude this synthesis by drawing together the strands that compose a complete garment of ethics. This sums up the proposal for a new system of ethics which has formed the basis for this study.

A summary statement must first answer the question of why an ethic must include the aforementioned dimensions. In the first place, I assume a normative view of reality, which holds that ethics must seek that our will resonate with three realities: what was intended to be, what by nature is, and what is forthcoming or what could be. Put another way, ethics must respond to what has happened to us, what is happening to us, and what will happen to us. Reality as we know it embraces space, time, and eternity. These dimensions form the vortex of ethics. When reality is conceived in a way that embraces propaedeutic, purposive, and proleptic definition, such a multifaceted ethic is required. Second, a probe of the human personality or soul, that range of faculties and functions that makes humans distinctive, reveals the full cache of attributes mentioned. Indeed, a person is seen as whole and well only when all of these traits function harmoniously. Finally, the system proposed is set forth because moral choices in and of themselves seem to require such a range of items immediate, immemorial, and impending for satisfactory transaction.

What, in sum, shall the ethic look like? A coherent and comprehensive moral system which encompasses all of the elements just outlined will function in a background, middle-ground, and foreground manner developing within its structure axioms, principles, and action guides to direct behavior. In the more public, pluralistic forum the foreground approach will dominate. In policy deliberation we will move more to the middle ground. In the deeper reflection of a society about vision and underlying purposes, we will move to the background elements. The society will also need such fundamental work from the groups and associations whose task it is to formulate philosophies and ways of life, for example, churches and political parties.

At the metaethical level axioms emerge such as respect for life and acceptance of death from the biologic and theological vectors. Principles such as kindness and freedom emerge from the psychic and philosophical vectors. Guides for action such as "do not harm" emerge from principles like *ahimsa* (noninjury) and are grounded in axiomatic imperatives such as "alleviate suffering." The practical exhortation "help the poor" rises from the principle of beneficence, which in turn is grounded in the axiomatic doctrine of human identification in suffering. These and many other nuances of the new system have been elaborated in the preceding chapters.

In sum, we have outlined a fundamental moral worldview and a spectrum of illustrative perinatal cases built on the leitmotif of the reciprocity of suffering and helping. Extrapolated from this background is an intermediate body of principles: justice, the leveling of suffering, and beneficence (which is the amelioration of suffering) are examples. Practical rules such as informed consent and truth-telling attempt to diminish the weight of contrived suffering, since the suffering derived from life itself is quite sufficient. Practical rules in turn radiate from the principles. At the root of any system of philosophy (a thought world that purposes to explain reality) is some basic principle. For Hume it was plurality; for Bradley, mystical monism; for Whitehead, process. Our system has posited as its basic principles suffering, death, and transfiguration. These have provoked an ethics of identification, sympathy, and ultimate vindication. The moral world view set before you might be capsuled in words Bertrand Russell used to summarize the three convictions that shaped his life: the thrill of knowledge, the need for love, and the relentless suffering of humankind.

CONCLUSION

Our long and circuitous exploration of ethics now draws to a close. We have sought to paint a big picture, not to obfuscate ethics in bewildering complexity but in order not to exclude dimensions that are vital and often decisive. The book has sought to be true to our secular and religious moral heritage. Most treatises on ethics today concentrate exclusively on a secular or a sacred purview, completely neglecting the other reality. We have seized on the compelling issues of perinatality as our field of example. As I look back, the ethics of nativity and natality, the concrete issues from AIDS to abortion to abuse, have provided further justification for the comprehensive ethical theory proposed. If a providing grace and inner stamina holds up, I hope next to explore in the same clinical and conceptual manner the realm of human mortality.

Notes

Preface

1. Homer, *Iliad*, trans. Richard Lattimore (Chicago: University of Chicago Press, 1951), 9.146, cited in Ben Kimpel, *Philosophies of Life of the Ancient Greeks and Israelites* (New York: Philosophical Library, 1981), p. 29.

Chapter 1: Ecological Ethics of Heaven and Earth: Population Expansion

1. *Global 2000 Report to the President* (London: Penguin Books, 1982), 1.
2. Ibid., p. 3.
3. Ben Wattenberg, *The Birth Dearth* (New York: Pharos, 1987).
4. *Global 2000*, pp. 15, 17.
5. Ibid., pp. 13, 17.
6. René Dubos, *A God Within* (New York: Scribners, 1972), p. 37.
7. Margaret Sanger, *An Autobiography* (London: Dover 1939), p. 28.
8. Germaine Greer, *Sex and Destiny: The Politics of Human Fertility* (New York: Harper and Row, 1984), pp. 350ff.
9. Ibid., p. 358.
10. Thomas B. Littlewood, *The Politics of Population Control* (South Bend, Ind.: University of Notre Dame Press, 1977), p. 5.
11. Ibid., pp. 79–80.
12. Kazoh Kitamori, *Theology of the Pain of God* (Richmond, Va.: John Knox Press, 1965).

13. Japanese Organization for International Co-operation in Family Planning, *Bird's-Eye View of Family Planning in Japan* (Tokyo: JOICFP, 1982), pp. 10ff.

14. Pope Paul VI, *Of Human Life (Humanae Vitae): Encyclical Letter of His Holiness on the Regulation of Birth* (Boston: St. Paul Editions, 1968).

15. Anna Quindlen, "Baby Craving," *Life*, June 1987, pp. 23ff.

16. Kenneth Vaux, "The Vatican's Cry of Protest," *Chicago Tribune*, 20 March 1987, sec. 1, p. 19.

17. Ibid., p. 19.

18. Paul Ehrlich, *The Machinery of Nature* (New York: Simon and Schuster, 1986), pp. 17, 18.

19. Ibid., p. 18.

Chapter 2: Apocalyptic Ethics of Human Sexuality: Plague

1. Stephen Jay Gould, "The Terrifying Normalcy of AIDS," *New York Times Magazine*, 19 April 1987, p. 33.

2. George E. Curry, "More AIDS Help Urged for Blacks," *Chicago Tribune*, 22 July 1987, sec. 1, p. 5.

3. "AIDS: Statistics but Few Answers," *Science*, 12 June 1987, pp. 1423–25.

4. Gould, "Terrifying Normalcy of AIDS," p. 33.

5. "The AIDS Dilemma," *Chicago Tribune*, 6 September 1987, sec. 4, p. 1

6. Lawrence Altman, "Inherited Factor May Play a Role in Risk of AIDS," *New York Times*, 10 May 1987, pp. 1, 14.

7. Shailer Mathews, "Apocalyptic Literature," in *Dictionary of the Bible*, ed. James Hastings (New York: Scribners, 1930), pp. 39–41.

8. Paul Johnson, *A History of the Jews* (New York: Harper and Row, 1987), p. 2.

9. Ibid., p. 27.

10. *Oxford English Dictionary* (Oxford: Clarendon Press, 1933), 3:654.

11. Albert Camus, *The Plague* (New York: Time Publications, 1948), p. 268.

12. Peter Davis, "Exploring the Kingdom of AIDS," *New York Times Magazine*, 31 May 1987, p. 32.

13. Ibid., p. 34.

14. The American Medical Association, *Code of Ethics of the American Medical Association* (Philadelphia: Turner Hamilton, 1981), p. 2.

15. *Report of the Council on Ethical and Judicial Affairs Statement on AIDS*, 1 December 1986.

Chapter 3: Biologic Ethics of Attraction and Affection: Being Sexual

1. John Costello, *Virtue under Fire: How World War II Changed Our Sexual and Social Attitudes* (Boston: Little, Brown, 1985).

2. Paul Ramsey, *Fabricated Man: The Ethics of Genetic Control* (New Haven: Yale University Press, 1970), pp. 22–59.

3. Sigmund Freud, *Civilization and Its Discontents* (London: Hogarth Press, 1930), p. 17.

4. "High-Tech Motherhood Creates Social Rifts," *Chicago Tribune*, 26 July 1987, sec. 1, p. 14.

5. Konrad Lorenz, *Das Sogennante Böse* (Vienna: Schoeler, 1963); W. Wickler, *The Biology of the Ten Commandments* (New York: McGraw-Hill, 1972).

6. Peter Singer, *The Expanding Circle of Ethics and Sociobiology* (New York: Meridian, 1981), p. 159.

7. D. T. Campbell, "Social Morality Norms as Evidence of Conflict between Biological Human Natures and Social System Requirements," in *Morality as a Biological Phenomenon*, ed. Gunther S. Stent (Berkeley: University of California Press, 1978), pp. 67ff.

8. Edward O. Wilson, *On Human Nature* (Cambridge: Harvard University Press, 1978), pp. 121–22.

9. George Edgin Pugh, *The Biological Origin of Human Values* (New York: Basic Books, 1977), p. 248.

Chapter 4: Psychic Ethics of Autism and Attachment: Being with Child

1. Margaret Mead and Ken Heymon, *Family* (New York: Macmillan, 1965), p. 14.

2. Ted Morgan, "Voices from the Barbie Trial," *New York Times Magazine*, 2 August 1987, pp. 23–24.

3. Oliver O'Donovan, *Begotten or Made* (Oxford: Clarendon Press, 1985), pp. 1–2.

4. Erich Neumann, *The Origins of Consciousness* (New York: Harper and Bros., 1962), pp. 114–15.

5. A. Portmann, *Zoologie und das neue Bild des Menschen* (Hamburg: Rowohlt, 1958), p. 68.

6. Doris Peyser Slesinger, *Mothercraft and Infant Health* (Lexington, Mass.: Lexington Books, 1982).

7. Edward Z. Tronick and Tiffany Field, eds., *Maternal Depression and Infant Disturbance* (San Francisco: Jossey-Bass, 1986), p. 88.

8. Mario Jacoby, *The Longing for Paradise* (Boston: Sigo Press, 1980), p. 229.

9. Willard Gaylin, "Feelings," in *Powers That Make Us Human*, ed. Kenneth Vaux (Urbana: University of Illinois Press, 1984).

10. Martin S. Pernick, *A Calculus of Suffering: Pain, Professionalism, and Anesthesia in Nineteenth Century America* (New York: Columbia University Press, 1985), pp. 148ff.

11. O'Donovan, *Begotten or Made*, p. 9.

12. Ibid., p. 8.

13. Ibid., p. 13.

14. Ernest Abel, *Fetal Alcohol Syndrome and Fetal Alcohol Effects* (New York: Plenum Press, 1984), p. 246.

15. Veronika E. B. Kolder, Janet Gallagher, and Michael T. Parsons, "Court-Ordered Obstetrical Interventions," *New England Journal of Medicine*, 7 May 1987, p. 1192.

16. Ibid., p. 1196.

17. Fernand Lamaze, *Painless Childbirth* (Chicago: Contemporary Books, 1958), p. 11.

18. Ibid., pp. 60–61.

Chapter 5: Philosophical Ethics of Ending Life: Abortion

1. John Noonan, "The Experience of Pain by the Unborn," in *Abortion, Medicine, and the Law*, ed. J. Douglas Butler and David F.

Walbert (New York: Facts on File Publications, 1986), pp. 365–66.

2. Ibid., p. 367.

3. Don C. Smith Jr., "Wrongful Birth, Wrongful Life: Emerging Theories of Liability," in Butler and Walbert, *Abortion, Medicine, and the Law*, p. 181.

4. Ibid.

5. Daniel Callahan, "Abortion: Some Ethical Issues," in Butler and Walbert, *Abortion, Medicine, and the Law*, p. 341.

6. Bruce Buursuma, " 'Defend Life' Pope Urges in Farewell," *Chicago Tribune*, 20 September 1987, sec. 1, p. 1.

7. Callahan, "Abortion," pp. 342–43.

8. Michael Tooley, *Abortion and Infanticide* (Oxford: Clarendon Press, 1983).

9. H. Tristram Engelhardt, *The Foundations of Bioethics* (New York: Oxford, 1986); Joseph Fletcher, *Humanhood: Essays in Biomedical Ethics* (Buffalo, N.Y.: Prometheus Books, 1984), p. 53.

10. See Oliver O'Donovan, *Begotten or Made*, p. 51.

11. Lisa Sowle Cahill, "Abortion, Autonomy, and Community," and Michael Tooley, "Philosophical Perspectives," in *Abortion: Understanding Differences*, ed. Sidney Callahan and Daniel Callahan (New York: Plenum Press, 1984).

12. Cahill, "Abortion, Autonomy, and Community," p. 265.

13. Alan Donagan, *The Theory of Morality* (Chicago: University of Chicago Press, 1977), p. 229.

14. Louis Janssens, "Artificial Insemination: Ethical Considerations," *Louvain Studies* 8 (Spring 1980): 5–6.

15. Daniel Callahan, "Minimalist Ethics," *Hastings Center Report* 11 (October 1981): 19–20.

16. Engelhardt, *Foundations of Bioethics*.

17. Ibid., p. 111.

Chapter 6: Epistemic Ethics of Knowledge and Ignorance: Genetic Health

1. Marc Lappe, "The Limits of Genetic Inquiry," *Hastings Center Report* 17 (August 1987): 5ff.

2. Alasdair McIntyre, "Seven Traits for Destroying Our Descendents," *Hastings Center Report* 9 (February 1979): 5–7.

3. Leon Kass, *Toward a More Natural Science: Biology and Human Affairs* (New York: Macmillan Free Press, 1985).

4. Robert Gale, "Concerns Rise over Use of Tissue from Fetuses," *New York Times,* 16 August 1987, sec. 1, p. 116.

5. John Fletcher, *Coping with Genetic Disorders: A Guide for Counseling Clergy and Parents* (New York: Harper and Row, 1982), p. 116.

6. Joseph Fletcher, *The Ethics of Genetics Control* (New York: Doubleday, 1974), p. 32.

7. Kenneth Howe, Margaret Holmes, and Arthur Elstein, "Teaching Clinical Decision Making," *Journal of Medicine and Philosophy* 9 (1984): 219.

8. Jay Katz, *The Silent World of Doctor and Patient* (New York: Free Press, 1984), see esp. chap. 7, "Acknowledging Uncertainty"; Charles Bosk, *Forgive and Remember: Managing Medical Failure* (Chicago: University of Chicago Press, 1979); David Hilfiker, "Facing Our Mistakes," *New England Journal of Medicine,* 12 January 1984, pp. 118ff.

9. Bosk, *Forgive and Remember,* p. 23.

10. Hilfiker, "Facing Our Mistakes," p. 119.

11. Katz, *Silent World,* pp. 116–17.

12. Ramsey, *Fabricated Man,* pp. 29–39.

13. John Fletcher, *Coping with Genetic Disorders,* p. 127.

14. Hannah Arendt, *The Human Condition* (Chicago: University of Chicago Press, 1959), p. 222.

Chapter 7: Historical Ethics of Eugenics: Sterility and Surrogacy

1. Julian Huxley, as quoted in Daniel T. Kelves, *In the Name of Eugenics* (New York: Knopf, 1985), pp. 260–61.

2. John A. Robertson and Joseph D. Schulman, "Pregnancy and Prenatal Harm to Offspring: The Case of Mothers with PKU," *Hastings Center Report* 17 (August 1987): 23ff.

3. Plato, *Republic,* trans. B. Jowett (Oxford: Oxford University Press, 1942), p. 17.

4. Quoted in Daniel T. Kelves, *In the Name of Eugenics* (New York: Knopf, 1985), pp. 116–17.

5. Ibid., p. 118.

6. McIntyre, "Seven Traits," pp. 5–7.

7. Kass, *Toward a More Natural Science*, p. 48.

8. Ibid., p. 53; Ramsey, *Fabricated Man.*

9. "Surrogate Moms Fight the 'Slavery,'" *Chicago Tribune*, 1 September 1987, sec. 5, p. 1.

10. Kenneth Vaux, "Baby Making to Buy and Sell," *Chicago Tribune*, 6 April 1987, sec. 1, p. 13.

11. Karl Rahner, "The Problem of Genetic Manipulation," in *On Moral Medicine*, ed. Stephen E. Lammers and Allen Verher (Grand Rapids: Eerdmans, 1987), p. 384.

12. Ibid., p. 387.

13. Adolf Hitler, as quoted in Robert Lifton, *The Nazi Doctors* (New York: Basic Books, 1986), p. 22.

14. Joseph Fletcher, *Ethics of Genetic Control*, p. 16.

Chapter 8: Legalistic Ethics of Save-or-Let-Die Decisions: Imperiled Newborns

1. Kenneth Vaux, "Ethical Issues in Caring for Tiny Infants," *Clinics in Perinatology* 13 (June 1986): 447–84.

2. Robert Weir, *Selective Nontreatment of Handicapped Newborns* (New York: Oxford University Press, 1984).

3. Earl Shelp, *Born to Die? Deciding the Fate of Critically Ill Newborns* (New York: Macmillan Free Press, 1986).

4. Ibid., p. 42.

5. C. E. Koop and F. A. Schaeffer, *Whatever Happened to the Human Race?* (New York: Good News Press, 1978); R. S. Duff and A. G. M. Campbell, "Moral and Ethical Dilemmas in the Special Care Nursery," *New England Journal of Medicine*, 25 October 1973, pp. 890–94.

6. D. M. Feldman, "Abortion: Jewish Perspectives," *Encyclopedia of Bioethics* (New York: Macmillan, 1978), pp. 5–9.

7. J. R. Connery, "Abortion: Roman Catholic Perspectives, *Encyclopedia of Bioethics* (New York: Macmillan, 1978), pp. 9–13.

8. Kenneth Vaux, "The Danville Siamese Twins: Religio-moral Perspectives," in *Euthanasia and the Newborn*, ed. R. C. Macmillan et al. (Boston: Reidel, 1987), pp. 66–80.

9. G. Dworkin, *Darwinism, Free Will, and Moral Responsibility* (Englewood Cliffs, N.J.: Prentice-Hall, 1970); M. Siegler and A. Jonsen, *Clinical Ethics* (New York: Macmillan, 1982).

10. "Vatican Condemns Mercy Killings," *Chicago Sun Times*, 14 December 1983, p. 10.

11. Paul Ramsey, *Ethics at the Edges of Life* (New Haven: Yale University Press, 1978), p. 202.

Chapter 9: Theological Ethics of Graceful Release: Life-Threatening Illness and Death in Children

1. Jane Brody, "Twin Boys Are Separated in 22 Hours Surgery," *New York Times*, 7 September 1987, pp. 1, 8.

2. Jan Van Eys, "When A Child Suffers . . . " (Texas Medical Center, Institute of Religion, September 1987, unpublished paper).

3. Most medical research projects must now include a process of ethical reflection. Institutional Review Boards (IRB's) often embody this function.

4. Pierre Teilhard de Chardin, *On Suffering* (New York: Harper and Row, 1974), pp. 57–58.

5. The cruelty of Klaus Barbie at the Adieu orphanage in France was revealed in the 1987 trial. See "Barbie and the Children," *Newsweek*, 15 June 1987; also *New York Times Magazine*, 26 May 1987.

6. Jean Piaget, *The Child's Conception of the World* (London: Routledge and Kegan Paul, 1929), p. 3.

7. C. E. Koop, W. B. Kiesewetter, and R. C. Horn, "Neuroblastoma in Childhood (Survival after Major Jungival Insult to the Tumor)," *Surgery* 38 (1955): 272.

8. Tilden C. Everson and Warren H. Cole, *Spontaneous Regressions of Cancer* (Philadelphia: Saunders, 1966).

9. James Gustafson, *Ethics from a Theocentric Perspective*, 2 vols. (Chicago: University of Chicago Press, 1983–84), 2:279ff.

10. Mitchell Locin, "Mandatory Job Leaves for New Parents Debated," *Chicago Tribune*, 15 September 1987, sec. 2, p. 3.

11. "Disabled Musician Plays on Pope's Heartstrings," *Chicago Tribune*, 16 September 1987, sec. 1, p. 10.

12. Kenneth Vaux, "Anno Domini 1981: The Ayatollah and Apocalypse," *Christian Century*, 18 February 1981, p. 168.

13. Fazlur Rahman, *Health and Medicine in the Islamic Tradition* (New York: Crossroad, 1987).

14. Carter Lindberg, "The Lutheran Tradition: Medical History" (1983, unpublished essay), pp. 3–4.

15. Wolfhart Pannenberg, *Human Nature, Election, and History* (Philadelphia: Westminster Press, 1977), pp. 14–15.

Chapter 10. Eschatological Ethics of Safekeeping the Future: Child Nurture

1. Robert Jay Lifton, *The Nazi Doctors* (New York: Basic Books, 1986), p. 14.

2. Ibid., p. 468.

3. "Decline in Infant Deaths Slowing," *Chicago Tribune*, 17 September 1987, sec. 1, p. 6.

4. "For Children: A Fair Chance," *New York Times*, 6 September 1987, sec. E, p. 14.

5. "On the Death of Poor Babies," *New York Times*, 6 September 1987, sec. E, p. 14.

6. Ellice Lieberman, Richard Monson, Kenneth Ryan, and Steven Schoenbaum, "Risk Factors Accounting for Racial Differences in the Rate of Premature Birth," *New England Journal of Medicine*, 17 September 1987, pp. 743ff.

7. "Survie de l'enfant," in *World Health Organization* (Geneva: Statistics Volume, 1986), pp. 11–12.

8. Pan American Health Organization, *Epidemiological Bulletin* 4, no. 2 (1986): 1–5.

9. *United Nations Declaration of the Rights of the Child*, General Assembly Resolution 1386 (XIV), 20 November 1959, Supplement no. 16, p. 19.

10. Onora O'Neill and William Ruddick, *Having Children: Philosophical and Legal Reflections on Parenthood* (New York: Oxford, 1979), p. 155.

11. Ibid., p. 123.
12. "How Some American Catholics See John Paul II's Visit," *New York Times*, 20 September 1987, sec. 4, p. 28.
13. Wolfhart Pannenberg, *Theology and the Kingdom of God* (Philadelphia: Westminster Press, 1969), pp. 109–10.
14. Johannes Metz, *Theology of the World* (New York: Herder, 1969).
15. Otto Friedrich, "Non Requiescat in Pace," *Time*, 24 June 1985, p. 90.
16. Thomas Jefferson, *Notes on the State of Virginia* (1781–1785), Query XVIII, in *The Works of Thomas Jefferson*, ed. Paul L. Ford (New York: Lippincott, 1904), 4:17.

Synthesis

1. For a clear exposition of the traditional philosophical approach to bioethics, see Tom Beauchamp and James Childress, *Principles of Biomedical Ethics* (New York: Oxford, 1979).
2. See Alasdair McIntyre, *After Virtue* (Notre Dame, Ind.: University of Notre Dame Press, 1983).
3. See, for example, Gunther S. Stent, ed., *Morality as a Biological Phenomenon* (Berkeley: University of California Press, 1978).
4. In our time, the major theological work on the ethics of science and medicine is James Gustafson's two-volume, *Ethics from a Theocentric Perspective*.
5. Simone Weil, *Waiting for God* (New York: Harper and Row, 1973). p. 99.

Index